The Compendium
of Infection Control Technologies

First Workbook Edition, Book 1

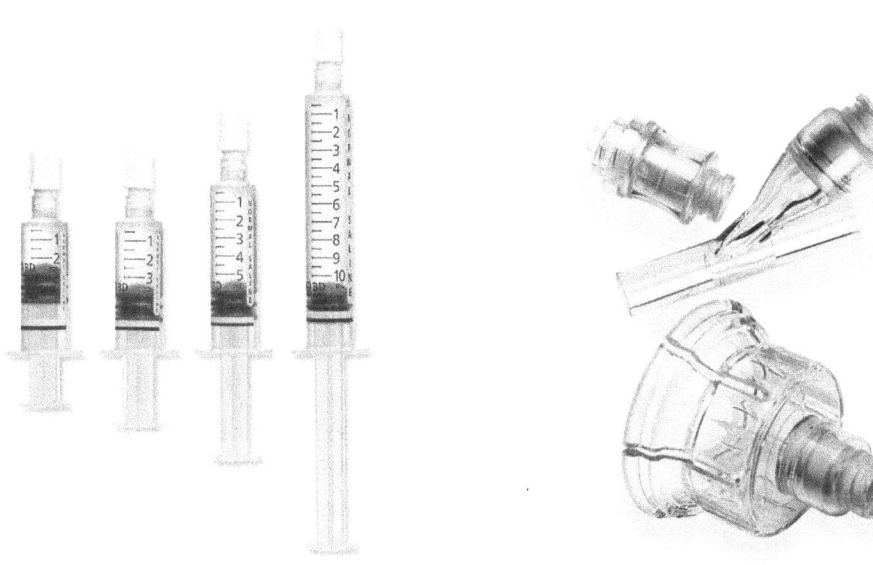

Consider the devices in this book and then order the literature and samples you need at:

www.MedicalSafetyBook.com

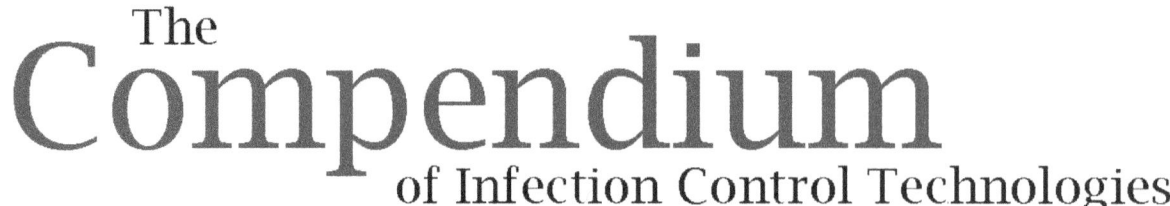

The Compendium
of Infection Control Technologies

INTRODUCTION

This workbook is designed to cut hundreds of man-hours off of the biomedical safety device evaluation portion of the task of creating an Exposure Control Plan.

In 2010, the incidence of needlestick injuries in the United States, alone, was about 384,000, as estimated by the CDC. Most needlestick injuries result from hollow bore disposable syringes and needles. Even though most needlestick injuries do not result in serious infection, they often inflict severe psychological damage on the injured employee. Waiting months or more after an injury, just waiting and waiting for one to find out if they have contracted HIV or one of the Hepatitis Viruses, can be devastating.

By using the proper safety devices, most of these injuries could have been prevented. The safe handling and disposal of needles and other sharp instruments must be a priority for all health care providers. This is not only to protect health care workers but to protect employers as well.

In the US, OSHA mandates that every employer, where even a single employee is at risk of possible exposure to infection via contaminated sharps, must have a written exposure control plan in place. As part of this plan, every engineering control and medical device designed to prevent such an incident must be evaluated for appropriateness for sharps injury prevention. The results of each evaluation must be maintained in written form and kept on the premises and made available to OSHA in the event of an inspection.

Why you should have your plan in place:

An Exposure Control Plan must be in place in every facility. Besides the obvious benefit of dramatically increasing employee safety, failure to have such a plan in place creates several major liabilities for health care facilities, all employers with at-risk employees, and of course, the employees. These liabilities include, but are certainly not limited to:

....Possible of sharps injuries

....OSHA actions in the event of an inspection. OSHA fines for failure to comply often rise to the level of six figures, sometimes 7 (really).

.... Employee legal actions that may follow an employee's sharps injury that could have been prevented, especially when there is an incomplete or no plan in place the might have prevented that accident.

Audit data suggests that of the occupational injuries that occur in hospitals, 16% are attributable to sharps injuries. (National Audit Office. The management of medical equipment in acute NHS Trusts in England, HCP 475 Session 1998–1999. London: Stationery Office; 1999. (Guideline Ref ID NAO1999).

As of 2003, it was estimated that needlestick injuries in the United States resulted in over 1000 Hepatitis B, Hepatitis C, and HIV infections in healthcare workers. Most, if not all, of these injuries could have been prevented.

All sharps injuries are considered to be potentially preventable. The preventability of such events are what puts the employer at risks. An employer who had ignored mandated procedures for sharps injury prevention would be in a poor position to defend itself from a lawsuit filed by an employee who had contracted a serious, or potentially lethal, injury, especially when they were using a non-safety device, rather than a properly evaluated safety device that could have potentially prevented the injury.

Can you afford a $100,000 fine?

OSHA requires that each facility seek out and evaluate all the medical devices on the market which are designed for the prevention of sharps injuries. The task is enormous and the fines for non-compliance often exceed $100,000. How often is often? In 2010, often was 164 times. Fines exceeding $100,000 were levied more than three times every week of the year.

Most of the devices that are listed in this compendium are currently available worldwide. Some may have already been discontinued or superseded. Let us know if you find either of these states to be true. More devices are available and our research is ongoing to provide you with access to additional devices as they become available. Updates to this publication will be made available at least once a year.

Best use of this publication:

After looking through each volume of this Compendium Workbook, you will need to choose which devices to evaluate. Go to MedicalSafetyBook.Com/signup.php and join for free.

Then click on the BROWSE SAMPLES link & order (usually free) samples of all of the devices you wish to pursue. Don't be shy; The manufacturers want to hear from you and give you the opportunity to choose their devices.

When you get your samples:

In your workbook, each safety device is paired with an evaluation form that will facilitate rapid evaluation of that device.   Look at the forms for each of the devices that you wish to evaluate. Make changes to the form if you feel you need to to make it conform to the specific needs of your facility. Use a different form if that works better for you. Email us if you need a digital copy of any of the forms so that you can revise it to conform to your facility's needs.

Printed version

This printed version is designed to be used as a safety device evaluation workbook. Once completed, the printed edition can be placed on your shelf to be presented to OSHA in the event of an inspection.

Please note, this notebook is only one part of your infection control plan and completing a thorough medical safety device evaluation and infection prevention plan, tailored to your facility's needs, remains your responsibility. No form will be perfect for every facility. Make changes to the forms and make them work for you.

This workbook is designed to replace many hundreds of man-hours of labor and many thousands of dollars of expenses that are involved in creating your exposure control plan.

If one nurse spent as little as two weeks working on this section of the ECP, it would cost, (with the average salary for registered nurses at about $40 per hour), it would cost about $3200. With this book, the savings would be more than $3000.00. And, by the way, it can't be done in two weeks. It can't be done in four weeks, either. Maybe 4 months. No, probably not.

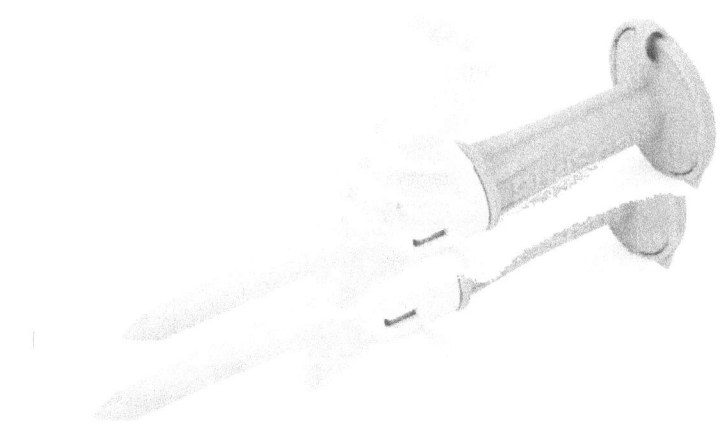

Table of Contents for Book 1

INTRODUCTION...2

TABLE OF CONTENTS FOR BOOK 1 5

JOEL'S DEDICATION...17

RON'S DEDICATION...17

ACKNOWLEDGEMENTS 18

    AOHP...19

    ISIPS...20

    NAPPSI 21

    PREMIER SAFETY INSTITUTE...22

FORMS FOR THE EVALUATION OF SAFETY DEVICES 24

    BLOODBORNE PATHOGEN EXPOSURE REDUCTION EVALUATION FORM....................................27

    BLOOD DONOR PHLEBOTOMY DEVICE EVALUATION FORM 29

    CATHETER SECURMENT DEVICE EVALUATION FORM 27

    DENTAL GLOVES 29

    SAFETY DENTAL GLASSES SAFETY FEATURE EVALUATION FORM 31

    SAFETY DENTAL SYRINGES 32

    DATE: DEPARTMENT: OCCUPATION:...32

    DISPOSABLE SHARPS CONTAINER EVALUATION FORM 35

    E.R. SHARPS DISPOSAL CONTAINERS...37

    FLUID TRANSFER DEVICE EVALUATION FORM 42

    GENERIC SAFETY DEVICE EVALUATION FORM...44

    GLOVES 46

    HOME USE SHARPS DISPOSAL CONTAINER 48

    I.V. ACCESS DEVICES...50

    I.V. CONNECTORS...52

    NEEDLE DESTRUCTION DEVICE EVALUATION FORM 54

    PATHOGEN EXPOSURE REDUCTION EVALUATION FORM 56

    REUSABLE SHARPS CONTAINER EVALUATION FORM 58

    SAFETY DRESSINGS 60

    SAFETY GLOVE EVALUATION FORM 62

    SAFETY SCALPEL EVALUATION FORM...64

    SAFETY SYRINGES 66

    SAFETY SYRINGES (AND SAFETY NEEDLES) 68

    SAFETY WINGED NEEDLE EVALUATION FORM 70

    SAFETY HUBER NEEDLE EVALUATION FORM 72

    SAFETY LANCET EVALUATION FORM..74

    SHARPS DISPOSAL CONTAINERS 75

    TUBES AND CONTAINERS EVALUATION FORM...78

    VACUUM TUBE BLOOD COLLECTION SYSTEMS 80

AMNIOCENTESIS TRAYS 82

    CURITY™ AMNIOCENTESIS TRAY 83

    SAFE-T-AMNIO™ TRAY 85

BLOOD COLLECTION EQUIPMENT 87

   CAPIJECT ® CAPILLARY BLOOD COLLECTION TUBES 89

   DEFENDER SAFETY NEEDLE HOLDER 91

   HAEMO-DIFF BLOOD SMEAR 93

   DONORCARE ® NEEDLE GUARD 95

   MAXIMUS BLOOD COLLECTION AND TRANSFER DEVICES 97

   MICROVETTE® CAPILLARY BLOOD COLLECTION SYSTEM 99

   MICROVETTE® CAPILLARY BLOOD COLLECTION SYSTEM 102

   MONOJECT ANGEL WING SAFETY BLOOD COLLECTION 104

   NEEDLE PROTECTOR 106

   PUNCTUR-GUARD BLOOD COLLECTION NEEDLES 108

   PUNCTUR-GUARD WINGED SET FOR BLOOD COLLECTION 110

   SAF-T HOLDER ® DEVICES 112

   SAF-T WING ® BLOOD COLLECTION SET 114

   SAMPLOK® SAMPLING KIT 116

   S-MONOVETTE® BLOOD COLLECTION SYSTEM 118

   VACUETTE ® QUICKSHIELD SAFETY TUBE HOLDER 120

   VACUETTE ® SAFETY BLOOD COLLECTION SET 122

   VANISHPOINT ® BLOOD COLLECTION SYSTEM 124

   VENIPUNCTURE NEEDLE-PRO ® DEVICE 126

CHAPTER BLOOD COLLECTION TUBES-PLASTIC 129

BLOOD COLLECTION TUBES –PLASTIC- 131

   MICROSAFE ® 132

   MICROVETTE® CAPILLARY BLOOD COLLECTION SYSTEM 134

   SAMPLOK ® TUBE BARREL HOLDER 136

   S-MONOVETTE® BLOOD COLLECTION SYSTEM 138

BLOOD SAMPLING SYSTEMS 141

   BLOOD DRAW HYPODERMIC NEEDLE-PRO ® DEVICE 142

   S-MONOVETTE® BLOOD COLLECTION SYSTEM 144

BLUNT TIP NEEDLES 147

   MONOJECT BLUNTIP 148

BONE MARROW COLLECTION SYSTEMS 151

   JAMSHIDI® BONE MARROW BIOPSY/ASPIRATION TRAYS 152

BONE MARROW TRAYS WITH SAFETY COMPONENTS 155

   MONOJECT™ BONE MARROW BIOPSY TRAYS 156

   SNARECOIL™ BONE MARROW BIOPSY TRAYS 158

NEWER DEVICES 161

   AIR BUBBLE REMOVAL DEVICES 162

   ALLERGY SYRINGES 162

   AMNIOCENTESIS TRAYS 162

AMPOULE BREAKER 162

ANESTHESIA TRAYS 162

APHERESIS NEEDLES 162

ARTERIAL BLOOD GAS SYRINGES 163

ARTERIAL CATHETER STABILIZATION PRODUCTS 163

ARTERIAL LINE DRAW 163

AUTOMATED FILLING OF IV SYRINGE DOSES 163

BIFURCATED NEEDLES 163

BIOHAZARD SPILL KIT 163

BLEEDING TIME DEVICES 163

BLOOD COLLECTION 164

BLOOD CULTURE BOTTLES 164

BLOOD CULTURE BOTTLE SAMPLE INTRODUCTION 165

BLOOD DONOR NEEDLES 165

BLOOD FILTRATION SET 165

BLOOD SLIDE PREPARATION DEVICES 165

BLUNT CANNULA NEEDLES 165

BLUNT SUTURE NEEDLES 166

BODILY FLUID WASTE DISPOSAL 166

BONE MARROW BIOPSY NEEDLE KITS 166

BONE MARROW COLLECTION SYSTEMS 166

BONE MILL, DISPOSABLE 166

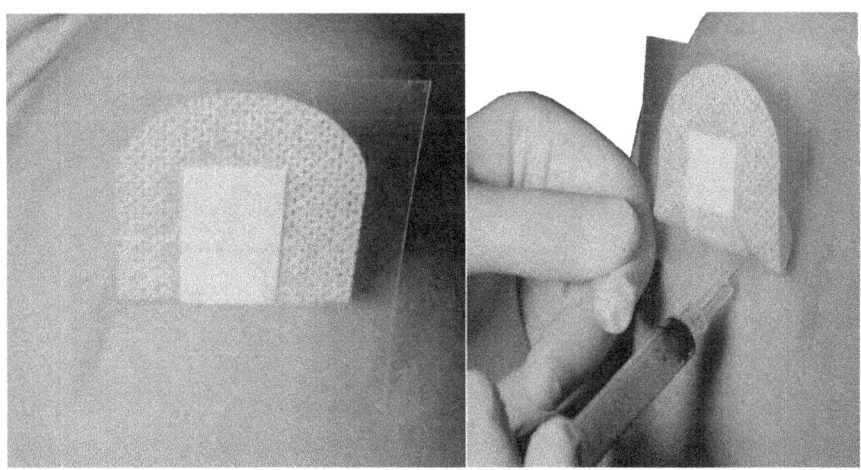

Categories of Devices

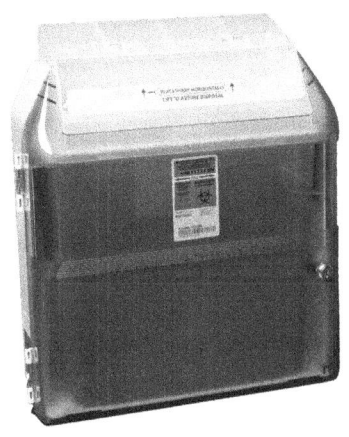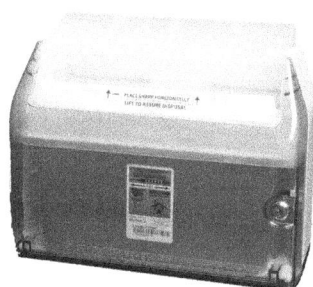

About 300 devices are included with the first 4 books of the workbook. The following is a list of the variouscategories of devices that are covered in the 12 sections of this workbook. Although you willprobably need all 12 sections and most, if not all of the categories.

Section 1

Introduction

Forms for the Evaluation of Safety

Devices Devices and Evaluation Forms

1. Amniocentesis Trays

2. Blood Collection Equipment

Section 2

3. Blood Collection Tubes - Plastic -

4. Bone Marrow Collection Systems

5. Bone Marrow Trays

6. Blunt Tip Needles

Section 3

7. Catheter Securement Systems

8. Closed System Protective Devices

9. Finger Protectors

10. Dental Safety Syringes

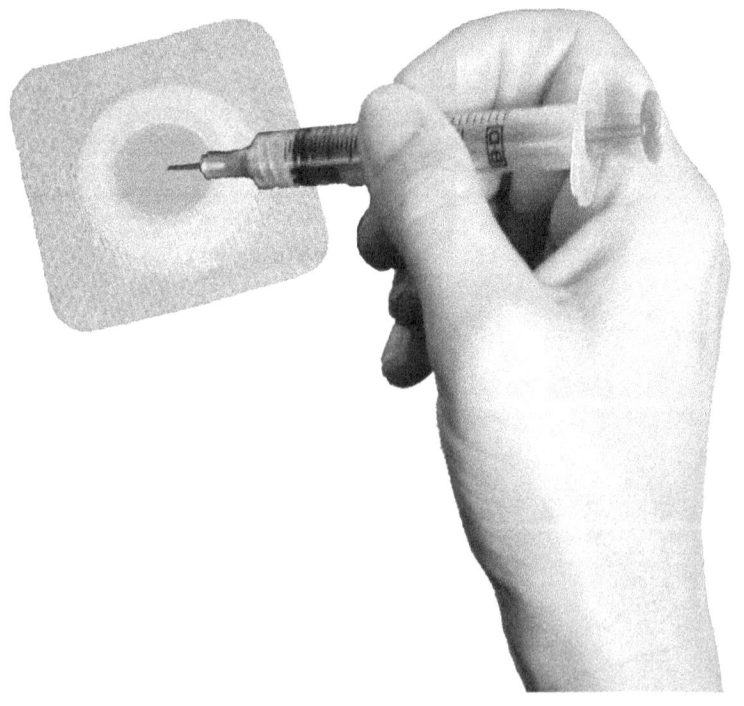

Section 4

11. Education and Training

12. Introducer Needles

13. IV Medication Delivery Systems

14. Laboratory Devices

15. Lumbar Puncture and Myelogram Trays

16. Masks and Goggles - Plastic

Section 5

17. Medical Waste Disposal Systems

18. Needle Destruction Products

19. Needle Disintegration Products

20. Needle-Free Drug Delivery Trocar

Section 6

21. Needle-free I.V. Systems

22. Needle-Free Injection Systems for Insulin

23. Needleless Jet Injection Systems

24. Needleless Transfer Devices

25. Needleless Urine Sampling

26. Needlestick Control Systems

27. Needle Recapper/Exchanger - 4-UP

28. Percutaneous Endoscopic Grastronomy Kits.

Section 7

29. Preemptive Dressings

30. Pre-Filled Syringes

31. Prep Razor

32. Regulatory Compliance

33. Retracting Needles

Section 8

34. Safety Arterial Blood Gas Syringe

35. Safety Capillary Blood Collection Systems

36. Safety Cord Blood Collection System

37. Safety Epidural Needle

38. Safety Huber Needles

39. Safety Instrument Transfer Drapes

Section 9

40. Safety IV Access Products

41. Safety IV Catheters

42. Safety Lancet

43. Safety Needles

44. Safety Picc Introducer

45. Safety Scalpels

Section 10

46. Safety Sliding Sheath Syringes

47. Spinal Safety Needles

48. Safety Suture Products

49. Staple Removal Devices

50. Safety Syringes

51. Safety Trays

52. Safety Winged Infusion Sets

Section 11

53. Safety Winged Set for Blood Collection

54. Scalpel Blade Remover

55. Scalpel Blades

56. Sharps Disposal Containers

57. Sharps Disposable Containers – Reusable

Section 12

58. Sharps Disposal Container / In-room

59. Sharps Retrieval System

60. Sharps Strainers

61. I.V.Catheter

62. Splash Protectors

63. Suction

64. Surgical Sharps Protection

65. Syringe Safety Trays

66. Thoracentesis Trays with Safety Components

67. Vial Adapters

68. Wound Closure Technologies

69. Wound Irrigation

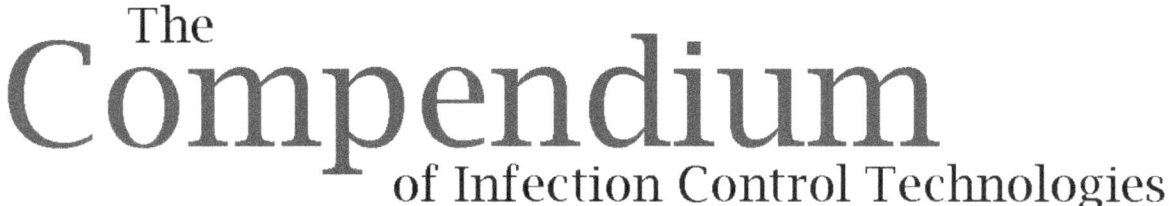

The Compendium
of Infection Control Technologies

First Workbook Edition Volume 1 - Book 1

The definitive guide to sharps safety andinfection control product evaluation

Published By Biomedical Safety Publishing, LLC

www.MedicalSafetyBook.com

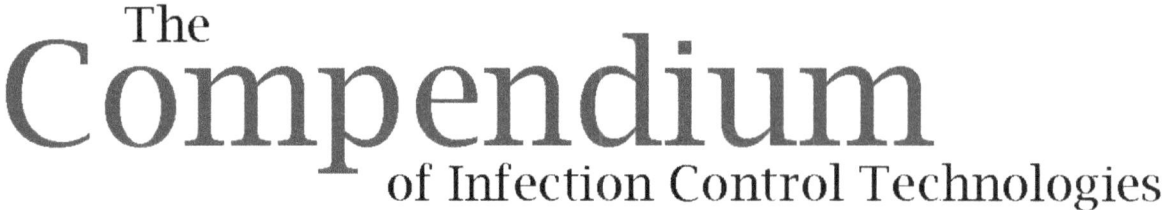

The Compendium
of Infection Control Technologies

Copyright Notice

Dedication

Joel's Dedication

This book is dedicated to my mom for giving me her brains; To my dad for giving me his temperament; To my ex-wifes, Ginger and Jan, for their patience and support and to my kids, Brent, Kirk, and Tylor for making life interesting and to the University of Missouri, School of Veterinary Medicine, for giving me a far better education than I could have ever imagined. And to my newest, my granddaughter, Elena..

Ron's Dedication

This book is dedicated to God for my wonderful life, to my kind and caring parents, to my loving wife, Melanie, and to each of my children and grandchildren.

We, Joel Rossen and Ron Stoker, wish to thank and acknowledge the organizations on the following pages for their unselfish assistance in the compilation of the Compendium and for graciously informing their members and subscribers about the availability of this publication.

We ask that you please look at their display pages and visit their websites.

Medical and Occupational Safety Organizations and Medical Infection Control Publications

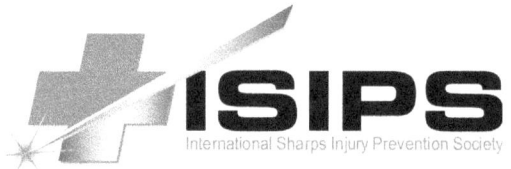

ISIPS
International Sharps Injury Prevention Society

NATIONAL ALLIANCE FOR THE PRIMARY

NAPPSI

PREVENTION OF SHARPS INJURIES

PREMIER

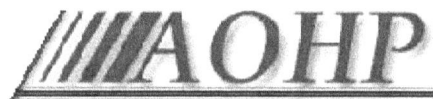

AOHP   Association of Occupational Health Professionals
in HEALTHCARE

Association of Occupational Health Professionals in HEALTHCARE

Mission: The AOHP is dedicated to promoting the health and safety of workers in healthcare.

This is accomplished through:

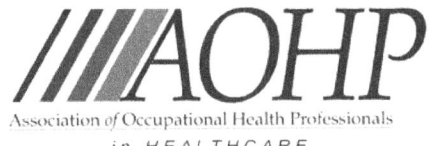

- Advocating for employee health and safety
- Occupational health education and networking opportunities
- Health and safety advancement through best practice and research
- Partnering with employers, regulatory agencies and related associations

Vision: AOHP will be the defining resource and the leading advocate for occupational health and safety in healthcare.

Legal and Ethical Issues

The occupational health professional has a legal and ethical obligation to protect the rights of the client and act as advocate to insure equal access to occupational health services. The occupational health professional is charged with the responsibility to provide a safe and healthful work environment for healthcare workers.

Rationale:

Collaboration with other health professionals and community health agencies are necessary in order to provide quality care and safeguard clients from unethic and illegal actions.

Objectives:

- 1. Safeguard confidential information in accordance with the law
- 2. Accept societal obligations as a professional and community member
- 3. Maintain individual competence in occupational health
- 4. Accept responsibility for individual judgments and actions
- 5. Identify and resolve ethical dilemmas
- 6. Provide uniform healthcare in the work environment for all healthcare workers
- 7. Promote collaboration with other health and community professionals

For information about our annual conferences, please visit our website www.AOHP.org or contact AOHP Headquarters.

Organizational Website:	www.AOHP.org
Organization:	AOHP Headquarters 109 VIP Drive Suite 220 Wexford, PA 15090 (866) 275-1366 info@aohp.org

Occupational Safety Organizations

ISIPS

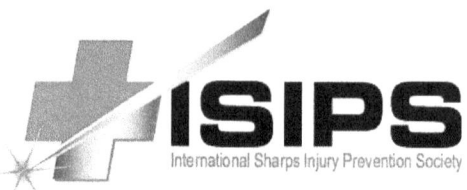
International Sharps Injury Prevention Society

Mission:
ISIPS believes that a significant number of needlesticks and other sharps injuries can be reduced each year. ISIPS promotes safety-engineered products and services that meet the goal of preventing percutaneous injury and exposure to bloodborne pathogens. In addition, ISIPS takes the most current information available and disseminates it to healthcare workers, infection control managers, and other interested parties. The ISIPS newsletters are issued weekly with information concerning sharps injury news, emerging sharps prevention products and technologies, the regulatory and legislative environment surrounding sharps injuries, and the latest information on HIV, Hepatitis, and other infection control interests.

Objectives: ISIPS promotes safety services and products that can reduce or eliminate needlestick and other sharps injuries.

We frequently conduct and promote a variety of activities that promote sharps safety. These activities include:

- Annual International Sharps Injury Prevention Awareness Month held in December of each year.

- Sharps Injury Prevention Award given to recipients that have made outstanding achievements in needlestick reduction each year.

- Participation in the Needlestick Prevention Tour seminars that provide outreach programs to state hospital associations, local APIC chapters, and large hospital systems.

- Provide presentations at national and international safety conferences.

- Provide articles for a number of infection control and clinician-focused medical journals.

- Provide continuing education on sharps safety and blood exposure prevention products and procedures. Presentations can be viewed at www.isips.org/prevention.html

Organizational website:	www.ISIPS.org
Organization:	ISIPS 10046 Prestwick Circle South Jordan, UT 84095 (801) 280 8797 Info@ISIPS.org

Medical Safety Organizations

NAPPSI

The National Alliance for the Primary Prevention of Sharps Injuries (NAPPSI) is a group of health organizations, medical device manufacturers, healthcare professionals, and others working cooperatively to reduce sharps injuries by reducing the number of sharps introduced into the healthcare workplace. Primary prevention means utilizing technologies and practices that either reduce or eliminate the need to use needles and other medical sharps. "No needle = No Risk"

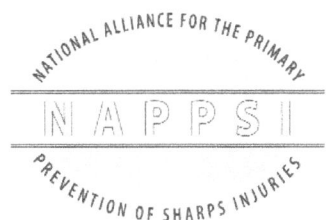

Examples of primary prevention technologies include:

- Catheter securement
- Laser technologies
- Needle-free infusion devices
- Non-needle wound closure
- Non-needle drug delivery systems

The goals of the Alliance are:

- To promote Primary Prevention as an essential sharps-injury-control method.

- To encourage federal and state legislators to include Primary Prevention language in pending legislation.

- To gain support for Primary Prevention among organizations and professional association.

- Highlight innovations in medical technology in the healthcare workplace.

- Provide education and outreach solutions to Alliance members and others.

Organizational website:	www.NAPPSI.org
Organization:	NAPPSI 1778 Callissia Court Carlsbad, CA 92009 (760) 525-4341 info@nappsi.org

Medical Safety Organizations

Premier Safety Institute

The Premier Safety Institute is part of Premier, Inc., a healthcare alliance of more than 1,500 leading not-for-profit hospitals and healthcare systems. Established in 1999, the Premier Safety Institute provides important information, resources and tools on patient, worker, product, and environmental safety as part of its mission to promote a safe, error-free healthcare delivery environment.

PREMIER

The Institute coordinates safety-related activities intended to appeal to a broad healthcare audience - from its own hospital and health system members and suppliers, to national organizations and the industry at large.

Premier offers comparative databases and tools for quality and safety performance improvement. The Centers for Medicare and Medicaid Services (CMS) recently partnered with the alliance in a three-year quality incentive demonstration project through which participating and eligible hospitals using Premier's Perspective Online ™ database receive recognition and additional Medicare payment when they meet or exceed specific quality measures.

Visit the Premier Safety Institute's publicly accessible Web site at *www.premierinc.com/safety*, and:

- Subscribe online to *Safety Share*, the Institute's monthly online newsletter, and join more than 30,000 readers, many of whom are active safety practitioners.
- Browse our on-line Safety Store, which offers many complimentary items for download.
- Review comprehensive topic summaries and download documents, tools, slides, case studies and sample policies on key issues in safety, including:
  - Back injury prevention
  - Bar coding
  - Disaster readiness
  - Environmentally preferable purchasing
  - Infection prevention
  - Patient safety
  - Sharps injury prevention

Organization web site:	www.premierinc.com/safety
Organization:	Premier Safety Institute 700 Commerce Drive; Suite 100 Oak Brook IL 60523 630.891.4865 *gina_pugliese@premierinc.com*

Medical Safety Organizations

Forms for the Evaluation of Safety Devices

Forms for the Evaluation of Safety Devices

DISCLAIMER: Please note, this Compendium is not meant to be your entire Sharps Safety Program. You must evaluate not only the devices which are included below; you must also ascertain the applicability of this publication to your specific set of circumstances and your specific business. The authors will not be responsible for any failure on the part of the publication's users to complete a thorough Sharps Injury Prevention Program tailored to your business entity.

Below please find the complete set of forms that our device evaluation publication is based upon.

The forms in the e-book format are graphics only. If you click on them, a full screen image of the form will appear. For the purposes of your Sharps Injury Prevention Program, you are going to want a printable form that you can use to make your evaluations. While the following link will provide you with a full set of forms which you may choose to use with any devices that you evaluate that are not in this book, each of the devices presented herein are paired with a form and you can click and download the device description and its associated form for each of the devices.

Go to MedicalSafetyBook.com to download a printable set of evaluation forms if you need them.

This is a list of **the 28 forms** on the following pages

1) Blood-borne Pathogen Exposure Reduction
2) Blood Donor Phlebotomy
3) Catheter Securement Device
4) Dental Gloves
5) Dental Safety Glasses
6) Dental Syringe
7) Disposable Sharps Container
8) E.R. Sharps Disposal Containers
9) Fluid Transfer Device
10) Generic Form
11) Gloves
12) Home Use Sharps Disposal Container
13) I.V. Access Device
14) I.V. Connectors
15) Needle Destruction Device
16) Pathogen Exposure Reduction
17) Reusable Sharps Container
18) Safety Dressings
19) Safety Gloves
20) Safety Scalpel
21) Safety Syringes
22) Safety Syringes and Safety Needles
23) Safety Winged Needle
24) Safety Huber needles
25) Safety Lancet
26) Sharps Disposal Containers
27) Tubes and Containers
28) Vacuum Tube Blood Collection

Notice: All of these forms are copyright ISIPS, TDICT, or both.

Many of the forms in the following books will not display copyright notices because space on the pages has been preserved for your evaluation purposes. While copyright notices may not appear on the individual forms when they appear in the book, the copyright still applies.

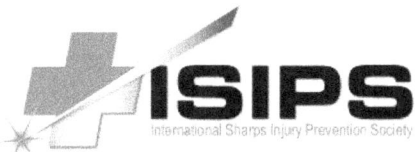

BLOODBORNE PATHOGEN EXPOSURE REDUCTION EVALUATION FORM

Date: _____ Department:_____

Evaluator: _____ Product: _____ Number of times used: _____

Please **circle** the most appropriate answer for each question. Not applicable (N/A) may be used if the question does not apply to this particular product.

		Agree.........Disagree
1	The use of the device does not require extensive change in technique from the use of a standard device.	1 2 3 4 5 N/A
2	This device provides a better alternative to traditional devices.	1 2 3 4 5 N/A
3	This device is no more difficult to use than traditional products and requires no additional time.	1 2 3 4 5 N/A
4	The device works well with a wide variety of hand sizes.	1 2 3 4 5 N/A
5	The device is easy to handle while wearing gloves.	1 2 3 4 5 N/A
6	The device can be used by either right or left handed clinicians.	1 2 3 4 5 N/A
7	The safety feature of the device does not cause interference with the procedure.	1 2 3 4 5 N/A
8	The user does not need extensive training for correct use of the product.	1 2 3 4 5 N/A
9	The product is suitable for a range of uses across a variety of patient populations.	1 2 3 4 5 N/A
10	The safety feature of the product is a passive feature; it requires no intervention on the part of the clinician to activate.	1 2 3 4 5 N/A
11	The user's hands are protected from a sharp at all times.	1 2 3 4 5 N/A
12	The device gives indication of safety feature activation (if one is added.)	1 2 3 4 5 N/A
13	The winged needle has an undefeatable safety feature that provides permanent coverage of the sharp.	1 2 3 4 5 N/A
14	The winged needle operates reliably.	1 2 3 4 5 N/A
15	The design of the product suggests proper use.	1 2 3 4 5 N/A
16	The use of the product reduces the risk of exposure to blood or other potentially infectious materials and therefore reduces the potential of exposure to bloodborne pathogens.	1 2 3 4 5 N/A

Of the above questions, which three are the most important to your safety when using this product?

Are there other questions which you feel should be asked regarding the safety features of this product?

Conclusions: _____

. _____

. _____

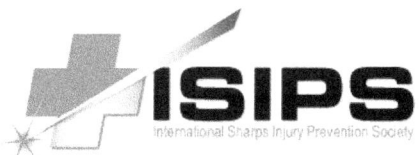

BLOOD DONOR PHLEBOTOMY DEVICE EVALUATION FORM

Date: _____ Department: _____

Evaluator: _____ Product: _____ Number of times used: _____

Please **circle** the most appropriate answer for each question. Not applicable (N/A) may be used if the question does not apply to this particular product.

		Agree.........Disagree
1	The safety feature does not obstruct vision of the tip of the needle.	1 2 3 4 5 N/A
2	This product does not require more time to use than a non-safety device.	1 2 3 4 5 N/A
3	Use of this product requires you to use the safety feature.	1 2 3 4 5 N/A
4	The safety feature works well with a wide variety of hand sizes.	1 2 3 4 5 N/A
5	The device is easy to handle while wearing gloves.	1 2 3 4 5 N/A
6	There is a clear and unmistakable change (audible or visible) that occurs when the safety feature is activated.	1 2 3 4 5 N/A
7	The safety feature operates reliably.	1 2 3 4 5 N/A
8	The needle is immediately shielded or retracted upon removal from vein.	1 2 3 4 5 N/A
9	The needle shielding is engaged from behind the needle.	1 2 3 4 5 N/A
10	After being placed in the permanently locked position the safety feature cannot be undone.	1 2 3 4 5 N/A
11	This safety product is no more difficult to use than non-safety products.	1 2 3 4 5 N/A
12	The user does not need extensive training for correct use of the product.	1 2 3 4 5 N/A
13	The design of the product suggests proper use.	1 2 3 4 5 N/A
14	It is not easy to skip a crucial step in proper use of the device.	1 2 3 4 5 N/A
15	The product can be easily used in either hand.	1 2 3 4 5 N/A
16	This device provides a better alternative to traditional blood donor phlebotomy devices.	1 2 3 4 5 N/A
17	The product is compatible for use with current blood collection sets produced by a variety of manufacturers.	1 2 3 4 5 N/A

Of the above questions, which three are the most important to your safety when using this product?

Are there other questions which you feel should be asked regarding the safety features of this product?

Conclusions:

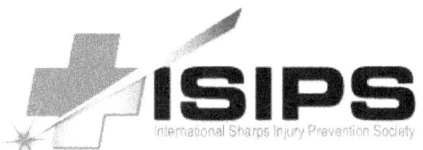

CATHETER SECURMENT DEVICE EVALUATION FORM

Date: _____ Department: _____
Evaluator: _____ Product: _____ Number of times used: _____

Please **circle** the most appropriate answer for each question. Not applicable (N/A) may be used if the question does not apply to this particular product.

		Agree.........Disagree
1	The product eliminates the need to use a suture needle.	1 2 3 4 5 N/A
2	The use of this product does not increase the number of needle sticks to the patient.	1 2 3 4 5 N/A
3	The use of this product does not interfere with the normal use of the catheter that it is securing.	1 2 3 4 5 N/A
4	The use of this product does not compromise safety features of catheter that it is securing.	1 2 3 4 5 N/A
5	The product does not require more time to use than suture or tape.	1 2 3 4 5 N/A
6	This device provides a better alternative to traditional catheter securement methods such as suture or tape.	1 2 3 4 5 N/A
7	This catheter securement device is no more difficult to use than traditional catheter securement methods.	1 2 3 4 5 N/A
8	The catheter securement device works well with a wide variety of hand sizes.	1 2 3 4 5 N/A
9	The catheter securement device operates reliably.	1 2 3 4 5 N/A
10	The device is easy to handle while wearing gloves.	1 2 3 4 5 N/A
11	The design of the product suggests proper use.	1 2 3 4 5 N/A
12	The user does not need extensive training for correct use of the product.	1 2 3 4 5 N/A

As part of this evaluation it is suggested that the following be reviewed:
OSHA Fact Sheet: Securing Medical Catheters -
http://www.osha.gov/SLTC/bloodbornepathogens/factsheet_catheters.pdf

Of the above questions, which three are the most important to your safety when using this product?

Are there other questions which you feel should be asked regarding the safety features of this product?

Conclusions:

SAFETY FEATURE EVALUATION FORM
DENTAL GLOVES

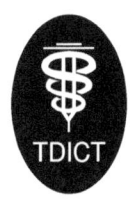

Date: _____ Department: _____ Occupation: _____

Product: _____ Number of times used: _____

Please **circle** the most appropriate answer for each question. Not applicable (N/A) may be used if the question does not apply to this particular product.

agree............disagree

1. The gloves dispense easily and quickly.. 1 2 3 4 5 N/A
2. The gloves are not discolored upon removal from the box.................................... 1 2 3 4 5 N/A
3. The glove **does not** have visible manufacturing defects (holes, etc)....................1 2 3 4 5 N/A
4. The glove is available for a wide variety of hand sizes.. 1 2 3 4 5 N/A
5. The size is easily determined after it has been removed from the box. (sizes are
    marked differently).. 1 2 3 4 5 N/A
6. The glove is easy to put on, even if hands are damp... 1 2 3 4 5 N/A
7. The glove retains appropriate sensitivity in the fingers....................................... 1 2 3 4 5 N/A
8. The glove protects the wrist securely.. 1 2 3 4 5 N/A
9. The glove is hypoallergenic.. 1 2 3 4 5 N/A
10. No excess powder remains afer removing the glove.. 1 2 3 4 5 N/A
11. The glove is comfortable for extended use... 1 2 3 4 5 N/A
12. The glove is easily removed.. 1 2 3 4 5 N/A
13. The glove allows the user to manipulate objects... 1 2 3 4 5 N/A
14. The glove **does not** tear when it contacts sharp edges of teeth, restorations, or
    ortho brackets.. 1 2 3 4 5 N/A
15. The glove **does not** become slippery on contact with saliva.................................. 1 2 3 4 5 N/A
16. Over gloves are easily donned removed.. 1 2 3 4 5 N/A
17. The glove **does not** have an unusual taste or odor to which patients object.......... 1 2 3 4 5 N/A

Of the above questions, which three are the most important to **your** safety when using this product?

Are there other questions which you feel should be asked regarding the safety/ utility of this product?

© June1993, revised August 1998
Training for Development of Innovative Control Technology Project

Safety Feature Evaluation Form
DENTAL SAFETY GLASSES

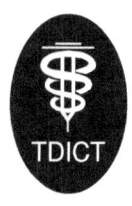

Date: _____ Department: _____ Occupation: _____

Product: _____ Number of times used: _____

Please **circle** the most appropriate answer for each question. Not applicable (N/A) may be used if the question does not apply to this particular product.

		agree............disagree
1.	The product **does not** fog up..	1 2 3 4 5 N/A
2.	The product works well with a variety of head sizes.................................	1 2 3 4 5 N/A
3.	The product is light weight..	1 2 3 4 5 N/A
4.	The product **does not** distort vision..	1 2 3 4 5 N/A
5.	The product is comfortable to wear for extended periods of time............................	1 2 3 4 5 N/A
6.	The product can be used while wearing presecription glasses............................	1 2 3 4 5 N/A
7.	The product can be used while wearing loupes..	1 2 3 4 5 N/A
8.	The product offers side protection...	1 2 3 4 5 N/A

Of the above questions, which three are the most important to **your** safety when using this product?

Are there other questions which you feel should be asked regarding the safety/ utility of this product?

© June1993, revised August 1998
Training for Development of Innovative Control Technology Project

SAFETY FEATURE EVALUATION FORM
SAFETY DENTAL SYRINGES

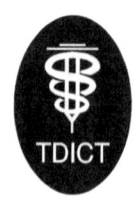

Date: _____ Department: _____ Occupation: _____

Product: _____ Number of times used: _____

Please **circle** the most appropriate answer for each question. Not applicable (N/A) may be used if the question does not apply to this particular product.

agree............disagree

1. The safety feature can be activated using a one-handed technique.......................... 1 2 3 4 5 N/A
2. The safety feature **does not** obstruct vision of the tip of the sharp and the intraoral injection site.. 1 2 3 4 5 N/A
3. Use of this product requires you to use the safety feature.. 1 2 3 4 5 N/A
4. This product **does not** require more time to use than a non-safety device............... 1 2 3 4 5 N/A
5. The safety feature works well with a wide variety of hand sizes.............................. 1 2 3 4 5 N/A
6. The device is easy to handle while wearing gloves... 1 2 3 4 5 N/A
7. The device is easy to handle when wet.. 1 2 3 4 5 N/A
8. This device accepts standard anesthetic carpules and does not hinder carpule changing.. 1 2 3 4 5 N/A
9. The safety feature **does not** restrict visability of carpule contents intraorally............ 1 2 3 4 5 N/A
10. This device accepts standard dental needles of all common lengths and gauges, and does not interfere with needle changing.. 1 2 3 4 5 N/A
11. The device provides a better alternative to traditional recapping........................... 1 2 3 4 5 N/A
12. Sterilization of this device is as easy as a standard dental syringe.......................... 1 2 3 4 5 N/A
13. *For syringes with integral needles only:* The needle on this syringe **will not** break while bending and repositioning in the tissue... 1 2 3 4 5 N/A
14. This device is no more difficult to break down after use for sterilization than a standard dental syringe... 1 2 3 4 5 N/A
15. The safety feature operates reliably.. 1 2 3 4 5 N/A
16. The exposed sharp is permanently blunted or covered after use and prior to disposal.. 1 2 3 4 5 N/A
17. There is a clear and unmistakable change (either visible or audible) that occurs when the safety feature is activated...1 2 3 4 5 N/A
    1 2 3 4 5 N/A
18. The user **does not** need extensive training to operate the product correctly.............1 2 3 4 5 N/A
19. The design of the device allows for easy removal of the needle from the syringe.....
20. The design of the device allows for easy removal of the carpule from the syringe.... 1 2 3 4 5 N/A

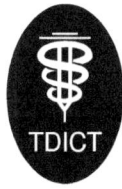

agree............disagree

21. The design **does not** entail excessive packaging or other excessive disposable items... 1 2 3 4 5 N/A

22. Removal of the needle from the syringe does not expose the operator to unnecesary risk.. 1 2 3 4 5 N/A

23. If the "scoop technique" is necessary, the design does not interfere or make the scoop more difficult. .... 1 2 3 4 5 N/A

24. The design eliminates the need for the "scoop technique."....................................... 1 2 3 4 5 N/A

25. The needle can be safely disposed of after recapping, without additional operator exposure to the needle.. 1 2 3 4 5 N/A

26. The safety feature is disposed of with the needle itself... 1 2 3 4 5 N/A

Of the above questions, which three are the most important to **your** safety when using this product?

Are there other questions which you feel should be asked regarding the safety/ utility of this product?

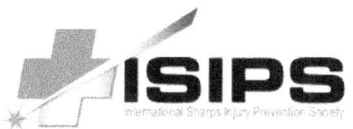

DISPOSABLE SHARPS CONTAINER EVALUATION FORM

Date: _____ Department: _____
Occupation: _____ Product: _____ Number of times used: ____

Please **circle** the most appropriate answer for each question.
Not applicable (N/A) may be used if the question does not apply to this particular product.

The Disposable Sharps Container:	Agree.........Disagree
1 Is puncture-resistant as certified to ASTM: F 2132-01.	1 2 3 4 5 N/A
2 Has documented compliance with Federal, State and local regulations.	1 2 3 4 5 N/A
3 Is leakproof on sides and bottom and during handling, storage and transport.	1 2 3 4 5 N/A
4 Is clearly labeled or color coded in accord with OSHA Bloodborne Pathogen (BBP) Standard.	1 2 3 4 5 N/A
5 Has a self-explanatory purpose & design, easily understood by busy users.	
6 Allows single-handed sharps deposit from all desired directions.	1 2 3 4 5 N/A
7 Can be placed at appropriate height allowing clear view of access by user.	1 2 3 4 5 N/A
8 Can be placed as close as feasible to where sharps are used.	1 2 3 4 5 N/A
9 Does not incorporate the use of needle unwinders which is prohibited by OSHA guidelines.	1 2 3 4 5 N/A
10 Is capable of taking and holding the size and volume of sharps used.	1 2 3 4 5 N/A
11 Permits safe, simple, entanglement-free disposal of sharps.	1 2 3 4 5 N/A
12 Is available in special designs for specific environments (Labs, OR, ER, etc).	1 2 3 4 5 N/A
13 Has an easily observable fill-status indicator, visible prior to sharps disposal.	1 2 3 4 5 N/A
14 Is stable when placed on horizontal surfaces in accord with product labelling.	1 2 3 4 5 N/A
15 Is designed to prevent hands or fingers from entering the container.	1 2 3 4 5 N/A
16 Defeats waste removal when open.	1 2 3 4 5 N/A
17 Has access designed to minimize sharps bounce-out.	1 2 3 4 5 N/A
18 Is designed so as to minimize risk of overfilling.	1 2 3 4 5 N/A
19 Has a closure mechanism that will not allow sharps injury during engagement.	1 2 3 4 5 N/A
20 Is resistant to manual opening when final closure mechanism is engaged.	1 2 3 4 5 N/A
21 Has optional locking bracketry.	1 2 3 4 5 N/A
22 Is easy to assemble, if required, and product is easily stored/stacked	1 2 3 4 5 N/A
23 Has rugged mounting brackets that are easy to service and decontaminate.	1 2 3 4 5 N/A
24 The design of the product is intuitive and does not require extensive user training.	1 2 3 4 5 N/A
25 Has a handle above the fill line that allows safe carrying of full container.	1 2 3 4 5 N/A
26 Is autoclavable, if necessary.	1 2 3 4 5 N/A
27 Has a design and final disposal that is environmentally sound.	1 2 3 4 5 N/A

Additional Evaluator concerns or comments:_____
_____

SAFETY FEATURE EVALUATION FORM
E. R. SHARPS DISPOSAL CONTAINERS

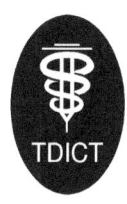

Date: _____ Department: _____ Occupation: _____

Product: _____ Number of times used: _____

Please **circle** the most appropriate answer for each question. Not applicable (N/A) may be used if the question does not apply to this particular product.

agree............disagree

1. The container's shape, its markings, or its color, imply danger which can be understood by visitors, children, and patients.. 1 2 3 4 5 N/A
2. The implied warning of danger can be seen from the angle at which people commonly view it. (very short people, people in wheel chairs, children, etc.)........... 1 2 3 4 5 N/A
3. The container can be placed in a location that is easily accessible during emergency procedures. ....1 2 3 4 5 N/A
4. The container's purpose is self-explanatory and easily understood by a worker who may be pressed for time or unfamiliar with the hospital setting....................... 1 2 3 4 5 N/A
5. The container can accept sharps from any direction desired................................. 1 2 3 4 5 N/A
6. The container can accept all sizes and shapes of sharps.....................................1 2 3 4 5 N/A
7. The container is temporarily closeable, and will not spill contents (even after being dropped down a flight of stairs).. 1 2 3 4 5 N/A
8. The container allows single handed operation. (Only the hand holding the sharp should be near the container opening.).. 1 2 3 4 5 N/A
9. It is difficult to reach in and remove a sharp. ....1 2 3 4 5 N/A
10. Sharps can go into the container without getting caught on the opening or any molded shapes in the interior..1 2 3 4 5 N/A
11. The container can be placed within arm's reach... 1 2 3 4 5 N/A
12. The container is puncture resistant... 1 2 3 4 5 N/A
13. When the container is dropped or turned upside down (even before it is permanently closed) sharps stay inside.. 1 2 3 4 5 N/A
14. The user can determine easily, from various viewing angles, when the container is full.. 1 2 3 4 5 N/A
15. When the container is to be used free-standing (no mounting bracket), it is stable and unlikely to tip over.. 1 2 3 4 5 N/A
16. The container is large enough to accept all sizes and shapes of sharps, including 50 ml preloaded syringes... 1 2 3 4 5 N/A
17. It is safe to close the container. (Sharps should not protrude into the path of hands attempting to close the container.)... 1 2 3 4 5 N/A
18. The container closes securely under all circumstances... 1 2 3 4 5 N/A
19. The product has handles which allow you to safely transport a full container........... 1 2 3 4 5 N/A
20. The product **does not** require extensive training to operate correctly..................... 1 2 3 4 5 N/A

Of the above questions, which three are the most important to **your** safety when using this product?

Are there other questions which you feel should be asked regarding the safety/ utility of this product?

© June1993, revised August 1998
Training for Development of Innovative Control Technology Project

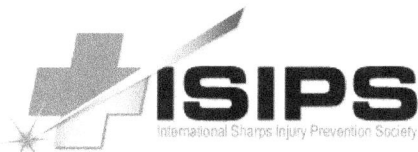

FLUID TRANSFER DEVICE EVALUATION FORM

Date: _____ Department: _____

Evaluator: _____ Product: _____ Number of times used: _____

Please **circle** the most appropriate answer for each question. Not applicable (N/A) may be used if the question does not apply to this particular product.

		Agree.........Disagree
1	The use of the fluid transfer device does not require extensive change in technique from the use of standard products.	1 2 3 4 5 N/A
2	This device provides a better alternative to traditional products.	1 2 3 4 5 N/A
3	This device is no more difficult to use than traditional needles and requires no additional time.	1 2 3 4 5 N/A
4	The device works well with a wide variety of hand sizes.	1 2 3 4 5 N/A
5	The device is easy to handle while wearing gloves.	1 2 3 4 5 N/A
6	The device can be used by either right or left handed clinicians.	1 2 3 4 5 N/A
7	The safety feature of the device does not cause interference with the procedure.	1 2 3 4 5 N/A
8	The user does not need extensive training for correct use of the product.	1 2 3 4 5 N/A
9	The product is suitable for a range of uses across a variety of patient populations.	1 2 3 4 5 N/A
10	The e product removes a sharp from the procedure thus reducing the potential of a sharps injury.	1 2 3 4 5 N/A
11	The user's hands are protected from a sharp at all times.	1 2 3 4 5 N/A
12	The design of the product suggests proper use.	1 2 3 4 5 N/A
13	Use of the product requires you to use the safety feature.	1 2 3 4 5 N/A

Of the above questions, which three are the most important to your safety when using this product?

Are there other questions which you feel should be asked regarding the safety features of this product?

Conclusions:_____

_____

_____

_____

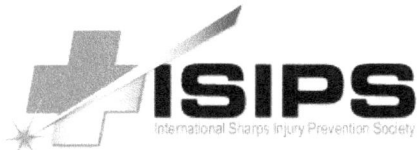

GENERIC SAFETY DEVICE EVALUATION FORM

Date: _____ Department: _____

Evaluator: _____ Product: _____ Number of times used: _____

Please **circle** the most appropriate answer for each question. Not applicable (N/A) may be used if the question does not apply to this particular product.

		Agree.........Disagree
1	The use of the device does not require extensive change in technique.	1 2 3 4 5 N/A
2	This device provides a better alternative to non-safety product.	1 2 3 4 5 N/A
3	This device is no more difficult to use than traditional non-safety product and requires no additional time.	1 2 3 4 5 N/A
4	The device works well with a wide variety of hand sizes.	1 2 3 4 5 N/A
5	The device is easy to handle while wearing gloves.	1 2 3 4 5 N/A
6	The device can be used by either right or left handed clinicians.	1 2 3 4 5 N/A
7	The safety feature of the device does not cause interference with the procedure.	1 2 3 4 5 N/A
8	The user does not need extensive training for correct use of the product.	1 2 3 4 5 N/A
9	The product is suitable for a range of uses across a variety of patient populations.	1 2 3 4 5 N/A
10	The safety feature of the product is a passive feature; it requires no intervention on the part of the clinician to activate.	1 2 3 4 5 N/A
11	The user's hands are protected from a sharp at all times.	1 2 3 4 5 N/A
12	The device gives indication of safety feature activation.	1 2 3 4 5 N/A
13	The device provides audible and visual feedback that the safety feature has been activated.	1 2 3 4 5 N/A
14	The device has an undefeatable safety feature that provides permanent coverage of the sharp.	1 2 3 4 5 N/A
15	The device operates reliably.	1 2 3 4 5 N/A
16	The design of the product suggests proper use.	1 2 3 4 5 N/A
17	Use of the product requires you to use the safety feature.	1 2 3 4 5 N/A
18	Use of the product removes a sharp thus removing potential for exposure to sharps injury and bloodborne pathogen exposure.	1 2 3 4 5 N/A

Of the above questions, which three are the most important to your safety when using this product?

Are there other questions which you feel should be asked regarding the safety features of this product?

Conclusions: _____

. _____

. _____

SAFETY FEATURE EVALUATION FORM
GLOVES

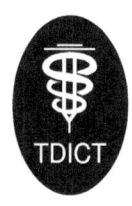

Date: _____ Department: _____ Occupation: _____

Product: _____ Number of times used: _____

Please **circle** the most appropriate answer for each question. Not applicable (N/A) may be used if the question does not apply to this particular product.

		agree............disagree
1.	The gloves dispense easily and quickly..	1 2 3 4 5 N/A
2.	The gloves **are not** discolored upon removal from the box...	1 2 3 4 5 N/A
3.	The glove **does not** have visible manufacturing defects (holes, etc)........................	1 2 3 4 5 N/A
4.	The glove is available for a wide variety of hand sizes..	1 2 3 4 5 N/A
5.	The size is easily determined after it has been removed from the box. (sizes are marked differently)...	1 2 3 4 5 N/A
6.	The glove is easy to put on, even if hands are damp..	1 2 3 4 5 N/A
7.	The glove retains appropriate sensitivity in the fingers...	1 2 3 4 5 N/A
8.	The glove protects the wrist securely..	1 2 3 4 5 N/A
9.	The glove **does not** damage the skin..	1 2 3 4 5 N/A
10.	No excess powder remains afer removing the glove...	1 2 3 4 5 N/A
11.	The glove **does not** tear through expected regular use...	1 2 3 4 5 N/A
12.	The glove is comfortable for extended use..	1 2 3 4 5 N/A
13.	The glove **does not** stick to tape...	1 2 3 4 5 N/A
14.	The glove allows the user to manipulate objects..	1 2 3 4 5 N/A
15.	The glove is easy to remove..	1 2 3 4 5 N/A

Of the above questions, which three are the most important to **your** safety when using this product?

Are there other questions which you feel should be asked regarding the safety/ utility of this product?

SAFETY FEATURE EVALUATION FORM
HOME USE SHARPS DISPOSAL CONTAINER

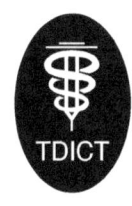

Date: _____ Department: _____ Occupation: _____

Product: _____ Number of times used: _____

Please **circle** the most appropriate answer for each question. Not applicable (N/A) may be used if the question does not apply to this particular product.

	agree............disagree
The container is puncture resistant...	1 2 3 4 5 N/A
The container is stable...	1 2 3 4 5 N/A
There is a handle which is robust, comfortable to carry, and compact...........................	1 2 3 4 5 N/A
The container allows single handed use..	1 2 3 4 5 N/A
The user can access the container from any direction..	1 2 3 4 5 N/A
It is possible to drop sharps into the container vertically......................................	1 2 3 4 5 N/A
Minimal or no force is required to put sharps into the container................................	1 2 3 4 5 N/A
The container opens and closes easily...	1 2 3 4 5 N/A
Container closure maintains integrity after repeated use.......................................	1 2 3 4 5 N/A
The box accommodates a range of sharps, including 12 cc syringe, butterfly, and lancet......	1 2 3 4 5 N/A
The size of the container is appropriate to its use...	1 2 3 4 5 N/A
No one (including a child) can access the contents of the container to retrieve a sharp......	1 2 3 4 5 N/A
Needles/tubing do not get caught on the opening or interior shape............................	1 2 3 4 5 N/A
There is a temporary lock for transport which is secure but reversible.........................	1 2 3 4 5 N/A
There is a permanent lock for final disposal which is not reversible............................	1 2 3 4 5 N/A
There is an absorbent lining to collect excess fluid..	1 2 3 4 5 N/A
The user can determine the fill level visually..	1 2 3 4 5 N/A
There is a signal when the box is 2/3 full..	1 2 3 4 5 N/A
The container is appropriately labeled...	1 2 3 4 5 N/A
Biohazard of container contents is apparent...	1 2 3 4 5 N/A
The box is not threatening to patients...	1 2 3 4 5 N/A
Use of this container in no way compromises infection control practices......................	1 2 3 4 5 N/A

Of the above questions, which three are the most important to **your** safety when using this product?

Are there other questions which you feel should be asked regarding the safety/ utility of this product?

SAFETY FEATURE EVALUATION FORM
I.V. ACCESS DEVICES

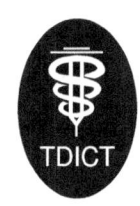

Date: _____ Department: _____ Occupation: _____

Product: _____ Number of times used: _____

Please **circle** the most appropriate answer for each question. Not applicable (N/A) may be used if the question does not apply to this particular product.

agree............disagree

1. The safety feature can be activated using a one-handed technique........................ 1 2 3 4 5 N/A
2. The safety feature **does not** interfere with normal use of this product.................... 1 2 3 4 5 N/A
3. Use of this product requires you to use the safety feature...................................... 1 2 3 4 5 N/A
4. This product **does not** require more time to use than a non-safety device.............. 1 2 3 4 5 N/A
5. The safety feature works well with a wide variety of hand sizes............................ 1 2 3 4 5 N/A
6. The device allows for rapid visualization of flashback in the catheter or chamber... 1 2 3 4 5 N/A
7. Use of this product **does not** increase the number of sticks to the patient...............1 2 3 4 5 N/A
8. The product stops the flow of blood after the needle is removed from the catheter (or after the butterfly is inserted) and just prior to line connections or hep-lock capping.. 1 2 3 4 5 N/A
9. A clear and unmistakable change (either audible or visible) occurs when the safety feature is activated... .... 1 2 3 4 5 N/A
10. The safety feature operates reliably... 1 2 3 4 5 N/A
11. The exposed sharp is blunted or covered after use and prior to disposal.............. 1 2 3 4 5 N/A
12. The product **does not** need extensive training to be operated correctly.................. 1 2 3 4 5 N/A

Of the above questions, which three are the most important to **your** safety when using this product?

Are there other questions which you feel should be asked regarding the safety/ utility of this product?

Safety Feature Evaluation Form
I.V. CONNECTORS

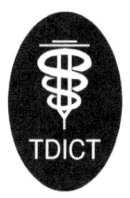

Date: _____ Department: _____ Occupation: _____

Product: _____ Number of times used: _____

Please **circle** the most appropriate answer for each question. Not applicable (N/A) may be used if the question does not apply to this particular product.

agree............disagree

1. Use of this connector eliminates the need for exposed needles in connections..... 1 2 3 4 5 N/A
2. The safety feature **does not** interfere with normal use of this product..................... 1 2 3 4 5 N/A
3. Use of this product requires you to use the safety feature...................................... 1 2 3 4 5 N/A
4. This product **does not** require more time to use than a non-safety device.............. 1 2 3 4 5 N/A
5. The safety feature works well with a wide variety of hand sizes............................ 1 2 3 4 5 N/A
6. The safety feature allows you to collect blood directly into a vacuum tube, eliminating the need for needles... 1 2 3 4 5 N/A
7. The connector can be secured (locked) to Y-sites, hep-locks, and central lines..... 1 2 3 4 5 N/A
8. A clear and unmistakable change (either audible or visible) occurs when the safety feature is activated.. 1 2 3 4 5 N/A
9. The safety feature operates reliably.. 1 2 3 4 5 N/A
10. The exposed sharp is blunted or covered after us ɔ and prior to disposal.............. 1 2 3 4 5 N/A
11. The product **does not** need extensive training to be operated correctly................. 1 2 3 4 5 N/A

Of the above questions, which three are the most important to **your** safety when using this product?

Are there other questions which you feel should be asked regarding the safety/ utility of this product?

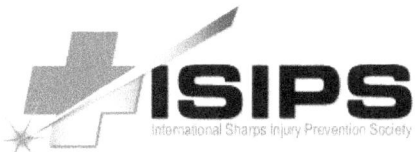

NEEDLE DESTRUCTION DEVICE EVALUATION FORM

Date: _____ Department: _____

Evaluator: _____ Product: _____ Number of times used: _____

Please **circle** the most appropriate answer for each question. Not applicable (N/A) may be used if the question does not apply to this particular product.

		Agree.........Disagree
1	The device destroys a needle and removes it from waste stream.	1 2 3 4 5 N/A
2	This device provides a better alternative to traditional needle removal processes.	1 2 3 4 5 N/A
3	The device is easy to use.	1 2 3 4 5 N/A
4	The device works well with a wide variety of hand sizes.	1 2 3 4 5 N/A
5	The device is easy to use while wearing gloves.	1 2 3 4 5 N/A
6	The device can be used by either right or left handed clinicians.	1 2 3 4 5 N/A
7	The user does not need extensive training for correct use of the product.	1 2 3 4 5 N/A
8	The product is suitable for a range of uses across a variety of patient populations.	1 2 3 4 5 N/A
9	The user's hands are protected from the sharp at all times.	1 2 3 4 5 N/A
10	The device provides audible and visual feedback that the safety feature has been activated.	1 2 3 4 5 N/A
11	The device operates reliably.	1 2 3 4 5 N/A
12	The design of the product suggests proper use.	1 2 3 4 5 N/A
13	Use of the product requires you to use the safety feature.	1 2 3 4 5 N/A
14	The device has an undefeatable safety feature that provides permanent coverage of the sharp.	1 2 3 4 5 N/A
15	The use of the device does not expose the user to other safety concerns.	1 2 3 4 5 N/A

Of the above questions, which three are the most important to your safety when using this product?

Are there other questions which you feel should be asked regarding the safety features of this product?

Conclusions: _____

_____

_____

_____

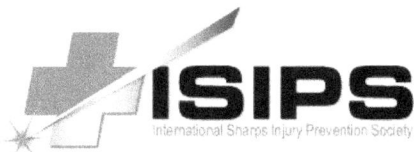

PATHOGEN EXPOSURE REDUCTION EVALUATION FORM

Date: _____ Department: _____

Evaluator: _____ Product: _____ Number of times used: _____

Please **circle** the most appropriate answer for each question. Not applicable (N/A) may be used if the question does not apply to this particular product.

		Agree.........Disagree
1	The use of the device does not require extensive change in technique from the use of a standard device.	1 2 3 4 5 N/A
2	This device provides a better alternative to traditional devices.	1 2 3 4 5 N/A
3	This device is no more difficult to use than traditional products and requires no additional time.	1 2 3 4 5 N/A
4	The device works well with a wide variety of hand sizes.	1 2 3 4 5 N/A
5	The device is easy to handle while wearing gloves.	1 2 3 4 5 N/A
6	The device can be used by either right or left handed clinicians.	1 2 3 4 5 N/A
7	The safety feature of the device does not cause interference with the procedure.	1 2 3 4 5 N/A
8	The user does not need extensive training for correct use of the product.	1 2 3 4 5 N/A
9	The product is suitable for a range of uses across a variety of patient populations.	1 2 3 4 5 N/A
10	The safety feature of the product is a passive feature; it requires no intervention on the part of the clinician to activate.	1 2 3 4 5 N/A
11	The user's hands are protected from a sharp at all times.	1 2 3 4 5 N/A
12	The device gives indication of safety feature activation (if one is added.)	1 2 3 4 5 N/A
13	The winged needle has an undefeatable safety feature that provides permanent coverage of the sharp.	1 2 3 4 5 N/A
14	The winged needle operates reliably.	1 2 3 4 5 N/A
15	The design of the product suggests proper use.	1 2 3 4 5 N/A
16	The use of the product reduces the risk of exposure to blood or other potentially infectious materials and therefore reduces the potential of exposure to bloodborne pathogens.	1 2 3 4 5 N/A

Of the above questions, which three are the most important to your safety when using this product?

Are there other questions which you feel should be asked regarding the safety features of this product?

Conclusions: _____

. _____

. _____

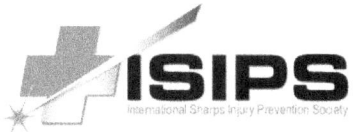

REUSABLE SHARPS CONTAINER EVALUATION FORM

Date: _____ Department:_____

Occupation: _____ Product: _____ Number of times used: _____

Please **circle** the most appropriate answer for each question. Not applicable (N/A) may be used if the question does not apply to this particular product.

		Agree.........Disagree
1	The Reusable Sharps Container is puncture-resistant.	1 2 3 4 5 N/A
2	The sides and bottom of the sharps disposal container are leak-proof.	1 2 3 4 5 N/A
3	The reusable sharps container is labeled or color coded red to ensure that everyone knows the contents are hazardous.	1 2 3 4 5 N/A
4	The reusable sharps container has a lid, and the container is maintained upright to keep liquids and the sharps inside.	1 2 3 4 5 N/A
5	The reusable sharps disposal containers can not be opened, emptied, or cleaned manually.	1 2 3 4 5 N/A
6	The reusable sharps container can be located as near to the area of use as feasible.	1 2 3 4 5 N/A
7	The reusable sharps disposal container does not incorporate the use of needle unwinders that are used to separate needles from syringes since this practice creates additional hazards and is now prohibited by OSHA.	1 2 3 4 5 N/A
8	The reusable sharps disposal container is of the appropriate size to accommodate the size and volume of sharps.	1 2 3 4 5 N/A
9	The reusable sharps disposal container has a prominent fill status indicator and provides the ability to see the contents of the container in order to determine the remaining capacity.	1 2 3 4 5 N/A
10	The design of the reusable sharps disposal container permits the safe disposal of sharps without snagging of sharps during insertion into the container.	1 2 3 4 5 N/A
11	The design of the reusable sharps disposal container prevents hands or fingers from entering the container.	1 2 3 4 5 N/A
12	The design of the reusable sharps disposal container prevents waste removal when open.	1 2 3 4 5 N/A
13	The design of the reusable sharps disposal container places handles above the fill line of the container in such a manner as to keep hands away from the opening during use of the handles.	1 2 3 4 5 N/A
14	The reusable sharps container has a safety closure mechanism that minimizes exposure to contents and injuries to the hand during engagement of the closing mechanism.	1 2 3 4 5 N/A
15	After being placed in the permanently locked position the safety feature cannot be undone.	1 2 3 4 5 N/A
16	The mounting brackets, if any, are rugged and provide ease of servicing and decontamination.	1 2 3 4 5 N/A
17	There is a permanent final closure so that once the sharps disposal container has been closed it is resistant to manual opening.	1 2 3 4 5 N/A
18	The reusable sharps disposal container can be placed in a secondary container if it cannot be sealed to prevent leakage.	1 2 3 4 5 N/A
19	The design of the product suggests proper use.	1 2 3 4 5 N/A
20	The user does not need extensive training for correct use of the product.	1 2 3 4 5 N/A

Of the above questions, which three are the most important to your safety when using this product?

Are there other questions which you feel should be asked regarding the safety features of this product? © 2005 International Sharps Injury Prevention Society – modeled after evaluation forms copyrighted by TDICT

SAFETY FEATURE EVALUATION FORM
SAFETY DRESSINGS

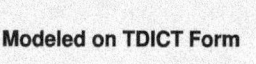

Date: ——————— Department: ———————————— Evaluator: ————————————

Product: ———————————————————————— Number of times used: ————————————

Please **circle** the most appropriate answer for each question. Not applicable (N/A) may be used if the question does not apply to this particular product.

DURING USE:
agree...........disagree

1. The safety feature can be activated using a one-handed technique...........................1 2 3 4 5 N/A
2. The safety feature **does not** obstruct vision of the tip of the sharp...........................1 2 3 4 5 N/A
3. Use of this product requires you to use the safety feature...1 2 3 4 5 N/A
4. This product does not require more time to use than a non-safety device.................1 2 3 4 5 N/A
5. The safety feature works well with a wide variety of hand sizes................................1 2 3 4 5 N/A
6. The device is easy to handle while wearing gloves.. 1 2 3 4 5 N/A
7. This device **does not** interfere with uses that do not require a needle.....................1 2 3 4 5 N/A
8. This device offers a good view of any aspirated fluid...1 2 3 4 5 N/A
9. This device will work with all required syringe and needle sizes............................... 1 2 3 4 5 N/A
10. This device provides a better alternative to traditional recapping............................. 1 2 3 4 5 N/A

AFTER USE:
11. There is a clear and unmistakeable change (audible or visible) that occurs
    when the safety feature is activated.. 1 2 3 4 5 N/A
12. The safety feature operates reliably.. 1 2 3 4 5 N/A
13. This device is no more difficult to process after use than non-safety devices........... 1 2 3 4 5 N/A

TRAINING:
14. The user **does not** need extensive training for correct operation........................... 1 2 3 4 5 N/A
15. The design of the device suggests proper use... 1 2 3 4 5 N/A
16. It is **not** easy to skip a crucial step in proper use of the device............................. 1 2 3 4 5 N/A

Of the above questions, which three are the most important to **your** safety when using this product?

——

Are there other questions which you feel should be asked regarding the safety/ utility of this product?

Based upon TDICT Evaluation Form

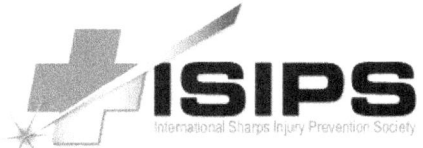

SAFETY GLOVE EVALUATION FORM

Date: _____ Department: _____

Evaluator: _____ Product: _____ Number of times used: _____

Please **circle** the most appropriate answer for each question. Not applicable (N/A) may be used if the question does not apply to this particular product.

		Agree.........Disagree
1	The use of the device does not require extensive change in technique.	1 2 3 4 5 N/A
2	This device provides a better alternative to non-safety product.	1 2 3 4 5 N/A
3	This device is no more difficult to use than traditional non-safety product and requires no additional time.	1 2 3 4 5 N/A
4	The device works well with a wide variety of hand sizes.	1 2 3 4 5 N/A
5	The gloves dispense easily and quickly	1 2 3 4 5 N/A
6	The gloves **are not** discolored upon removal from the box	1 2 3 4 5 N/A
7	The safety feature of the device does not cause interference with the procedure.	1 2 3 4 5 N/A
8	The user does not need extensive training for correct use of the product.	1 2 3 4 5 N/A
9	The glove **does not** have visible manufacturing defects (holes, etc)	1 2 3 4 5 N/A
10	The safety feature of the product is a passive feature; it requires no intervention on the part of the clinician to activate.	1 2 3 4 5 N/A
11	The user's hands are protected from a sharp at all times.	1 2 3 4 5 N/A
12	The glove is available for a wide variety of hand sizes	1 2 3 4 5 N/A
13	The glove is easy to put on, even if hands are damp	1 2 3 4 5 N/A
14	The device has an undefeatable safety feature that provides permanent coverage of the sharp.	1 2 3 4 5 N/A
15	The device operates reliably.	1 2 3 4 5 N/A
16	The design of the product suggests proper use.	1 2 3 4 5 N/A
17	Use of the product requires you to use the safety feature.	1 2 3 4 5 N/A
18	The glove retains appropriate sensitivity in the fingers.	1 2 3 4 5 N/A
19	The glove protects the wrist securely.	1 2 3 4 5 N/A
20	The glove **does not** damage the skin.	1 2 3 4 5 N/A
21	The glove **does not** tear through expected regular use.	1 2 3 4 5 N/A
22	The glove is comfortable for extended use.	1 2 3 4 5 N/A
23	The glove allows the user to manipulate objects.	1 2 3 4 5 N/A
24	The glove is easy to remove.	1 2 3 4 5 N/A

Of the above questions, which three are the most important to your safety when using this product?

Are there other questions which you feel should be asked regarding the safety features of this product?

Conclusions: _____

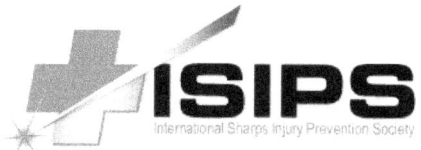

SAFETY SCALPEL EVALUATION FORM

Date: _____ Department: _____

Occupation: _____ Product: _____ Number of times used: _____

Please **circle** the most appropriate answer for each question. Not applicable (N/A) may be used if the question does not apply to this particular product.

		Agree.........Disagree
1	The safety feature of the scalpel can be activated using a one-handed technique.	1 2 3 4 5 N/A
2	The safety feature does not obstruct vision of the tip of the scalpel blade.	1 2 3 4 5 N/A
3	Use of this product requires you to use the safety feature.	1 2 3 4 5 N/A
4	This product does not require more time to use than a non-safety device.	1 2 3 4 5 N/A
5	The safety feature works well with a wide variety of hand sizes.	1 2 3 4 5 N/A
6	The device is easy to handle while wearing gloves.	1 2 3 4 5 N/A
7	This device provides a better alternative to traditional scalpels.	1 2 3 4 5 N/A
8	There is a clear and unmistakable change (audible or visible) that occurs when the safety feature is activated.	1 2 3 4 5 N/A
9	The safety feature operates reliably.	1 2 3 4 5 N/A
10	The safety feature has three positions: blade exposed, blade covered, blade permanently locked.	1 2 3 4 5 N/A
11	After being placed in the permanently locked position the safety feature cannot be undone.	1 2 3 4 5 N/A
12	This safety scalpel is no more difficult to use than non-safety scalpels.	1 2 3 4 5 N/A
13	The user does not need extensive training for correct use of the product.	1 2 3 4 5 N/A
14	The design of the product suggests proper use.	1 2 3 4 5 N/A
15	It is not easy to skip a crucial step in proper use of the device.	1 2 3 4 5 N/A
16	The product can be easily used in the right hand.	1 2 3 4 5 N/A
17	The product can be easily used in the left hand.	1 2 3 4 5 N/A
18	The product can be easily used in either hand.	1 2 3 4 5 N/A
19	The use of the product does not require passing scalpel with the blade exposed.	1 2 3 4 5 N/A
20	The handle is similar in size and weight to standard scalpel.	1 2 3 4 5 N/A
21	The scalpel handle has grips for stable handling.	1 2 3 4 5 N/A

Of the above questions, which three are the most important to your safety when using this product?

Are there other questions which you feel should be asked regarding the safety features of this product?

SAFETY FEATURE EVALUATION FORM
SAFETY SYRINGES

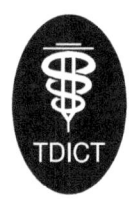

Date: _____ Department: _____ Occupation: _____

Product: _____ Number of times used: _____

Please **circle** the most appropriate answer for each question. Not applicable (N/A) may be used if the question does not apply to this particular product.

DURING USE:
                                                                    agree...........disagree

1. The safety feature can be activated using a one-handed technique...........1 2 3 4 5 N/A
2. The safety feature **does not** obstruct vision of the tip of the sharp............1 2 3 4 5 N/A
3. Use of this product requires you to use the safety feature............................1 2 3 4 5 N/A
4. This product does not require more time to use than a non-safety device.................1 2 3 4 5 N/A
5. The safety feature works well with a wide variety of hand sizes.................1 2 3 4 5 N/A
6. The device is easy to handle while wearing gloves.....................................1 2 3 4 5 N/A
7. This device **does not** interfere with uses that do not require a needle.......................1 2 3 4 5 N/A
8. This device offers a good view of any aspirated fluid................................1 2 3 4 5 N/A
9. This device will work with all required syringe and needle sizes.................1 2 3 4 5 N/A
10. This device provides a better alternative to traditional recapping...............1 2 3 4 5 N/A

AFTER USE:

11. There is a clear and unmistakeable change (audible or visible) that occurs
      when the safety feature is activated..1 2 3 4 5 N/A
12. The safety feature operates reliably..1 2 3 4 5 N/A
13. The exposed sharp is permanently blunted or covered after use and prior to dis-
     posal...1 2 3 4 5 N/A
14. This device is no more difficult to process after use than non-safety devices...........1 2 3 4 5 N/A

TRAINING:

15. The user **does not** need extensive training for correct operation............................1 2 3 4 5 N/A
16. The design of the device suggests proper use..1 2 3 4 5 N/A
17. It is **not** easy to skip a crucial step in proper use of the device.................................1 2 3 4 5 N/A

Of the above questions, which three are the most important to **your** safety when using this product?

Are there other questions which you feel should be asked regarding the safety/ utility of this product?

SAFETY FEATURE EVALUATION FORM
SAFETY SYRINGES (and safety needles)

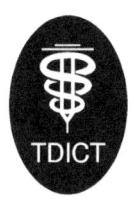

Date: —————— Department: —————————— Occupation: ——————————

Product: —————————————————— Number of times used: ——————————

Please **circle** the most appropriate answer for each question. Not applicable (N/A) may be used if the question does not apply to this particular product.

DURING USE:

agree............disagree

1. The safety feature can be activated using a one-handed technique............1 2 3 4 5 N/A
2. The safety feature **does not** obstruct vision of the tip of the sharp............1 2 3 4 5 N/A
3. Use of this product requires you to use the safety feature............1 2 3 4 5 N/A
4. This product does not require more time to use than a non-safety device............ 1 2 3 4 5 N/A
5. The safety feature works well with a wide variety of hand sizes............1 2 3 4 5 N/A
6. The device is easy to handle while wearing gloves............ 1 2 3 4 5 N/A
7. This device **does not** interfere with uses that do not require a needle............1 2 3 4 5 N/A
8. This device offers a good view of any aspirated fluid............1 2 3 4 5 N/A
9. This device will work with all required syringe and needle sizes............ 1 2 3 4 5 N/A
10. This device provides a better alternative to traditional recapping............ 1 2 3 4 5 N/A

AFTER USE:

11. There is a clear and unmistakeable change (audible or visible) that occurs
     when the safety feature is activated............ 1 2 3 4 5 N/A
12. The safety feature operates reliably............ 1 2 3 4 5 N/A
13. The exposed sharp is permanently blunted or covered after use and prior to disposal............ 1 2 3 4 5 N/A
14. This device is no more difficult to process after use than non-safety devices............ 1 2 3 4 5 N/A

TRAINING:

15. The user **does not** need extensive training for correct operation............ 1 2 3 4 5 N/A
16. The design of the device suggests proper use............ 1 2 3 4 5 N/A
17. It is **not** easy to skip a crucial step in proper use of the device............ 1 2 3 4 5 N/A

Of the above questions, which three are the most important to **your** safety when using this product?

Are there other questions which you feel should be asked regarding the safety/ utility of this product?

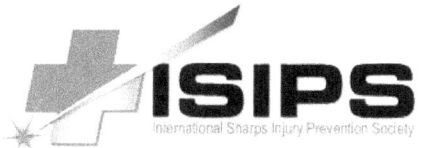

SAFETY WINGED NEEDLE EVALUATION FORM

Date: _____ Department:_____

Evaluator: _____ Product: _____ Number of times used: _____

Please **circle** the most appropriate answer for each question. Not applicable (N/A) may be used if the question does not apply to this particular product.

		Agree.........Disagree
1	The use of the Safety winged needle does not require extensive change in technique from the use of standard winged needles.	1 2 3 4 5 N/A
2	This device provides a better alternative to traditional winged needles.	1 2 3 4 5 N/A
3	This winged needle is no more difficult to use than traditional winged needles and requires no additional time.	1 2 3 4 5 N/A
4	The winged needle works well with a wide variety of hand sizes.	1 2 3 4 5 N/A
5	The winged needle is easy to handle while wearing gloves.	1 2 3 4 5 N/A
6	The winged needle can be used by either right or left handed clinicians.	1 2 3 4 5 N/A
7	The safety feature of the winged needle does not cause interference with the procedure.	1 2 3 4 5 N/A
8	The user does not need extensive training for correct use of the product.	1 2 3 4 5 N/A
9	The product is suitable for a range of uses across a variety of patient populations.	1 2 3 4 5 N/A
10	The safety feature of the product is a passive feature; it requires no intervention on the part of the clinician to activate.	1 2 3 4 5 N/A
11	The user's hands are protected from the sharp at all times.	1 2 3 4 5 N/A
12	The winged needle gives indication of safety feature activation.	1 2 3 4 5 N/A
13	The winged needle provides audible and visual feedback that the safety feature has been activated.	1 2 3 4 5 N/A
14	The winged needle has an undefeatable safety feature that provides permanent coverage of the sharp.	1 2 3 4 5 N/A
15	The winged needle operates reliably.	1 2 3 4 5 N/A
16	The design of the product suggests proper use.	1 2 3 4 5 N/A
17	The design of the safety winged needle allows it to be flush against skin without a high profile.	1 2 3 4 5 N/A
18	Use of the product requires you to use the safety feature.	1 2 3 4 5 N/A

Of the above questions, which three are the most important to your safety when using this product?

Are there other questions which you feel should be asked regarding the safety features of this product?

Conclusions: _____ -

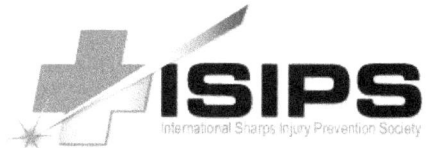

SAFETY HUBER NEEDLE EVALUATION FORM

Date: _____ Department: _____

Occupation: _____ Product: _____ Number of times used: _____

Please **circle** the most appropriate answer for each question. Not applicable (N/A) may be used if the question does not apply to this particular product.

		Agree.........Disagree
1	The use of the Huber needle does not require extensive change in technique from the use of standard Huber needles.	1 2 3 4 5 N/A
2	This device provides a better alternative to traditional Huber needles.	1 2 3 4 5 N/A
3	This Huber needle is no more difficult to use than traditional Huber Needles and requires no additional time.	1 2 3 4 5 N/A
4	The Huber needle works well with a wide variety of hand sizes.	1 2 3 4 5 N/A
5	The Huber needle is easy to handle while wearing gloves.	1 2 3 4 5 N/A
6	The Huber needle can be used by either right or left handed clinicians.	1 2 3 4 5 N/A
7	The safety feature of the Huber Needle does not cause interference with the procedure.	1 2 3 4 5 N/A
8	The user does not need extensive training for correct use of the product.	1 2 3 4 5 N/A
9	The product is suitable for a range of uses across a variety of patient populations.	1 2 3 4 5 N/A
10	The safety feature of the product is a passive feature; it requires no intervention on the part of the clinician to activate.	1 2 3 4 5 N/A
11	The user's hands are protected from the sharp at all times.	1 2 3 4 5 N/A
12	The Huber needle gives indication of safety feature activation.	1 2 3 4 5 N/A
13	The Huber needle provides audible and visual feedback that the safety feature has been activated.	1 2 3 4 5 N/A
14	The Huber needle has an undefeatable safety feature that provides permanent coverage of the sharp.	1 2 3 4 5 N/A
15	The Huber needle operates reliably.	1 2 3 4 5 N/A
16	The design of the product suggests proper use.	1 2 3 4 5 N/A
17	The design of the product allows for the viewing of the insertion site.	1 2 3 4 5 N/A
18	The design of the safety Huber needle allows it to be flush against skin without a high profile.	
19	Use of the product requires you to use the safety feature.	

Of the above questions, which three are the most important to your safety when using this product?

Are there other questions which you feel should be asked regarding the safety features of this product?

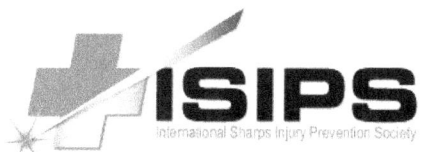

SAFETY LANCET EVALUATION FORM

Date: _____ Department: _____

Occupation: _____ Product: _____ Number of times used: _____

Please **circle** the most appropriate answer for each question. Not applicable (N/A) may be used if the question does not apply to this particular product.

		Agree.........Disagree
1	The use of the lancet does not require extensive change in technique from the use of standard lancets.	1 2 3 4 5 N/A
2	This device provides a better alternative to traditional lancets.	1 2 3 4 5 N/A
3	This lancet is no more difficult to use than traditional lancing methods.	1 2 3 4 5 N/A
4	The lancet works well with a wide variety of hand sizes.	1 2 3 4 5 N/A
5	The lancet is easy to handle while wearing gloves.	1 2 3 4 5 N/A
6	The lancet can be used by either right or left handed clinicians.	1 2 3 4 5 N/A
7	The safety feature of the lancet does not cause interference with the procedure.	1 2 3 4 5 N/A
8	The user does not need extensive training for correct use of the product.	1 2 3 4 5 N/A
9	The product is suitable for a range of uses across a variety of patient populations.	1 2 3 4 5 N/A
10	The safety feature of the product is a passive feature; it requires no intervention on the part of the clinician to activate.	1 2 3 4 5 N/A
11	The user's hands are located behind the sharp at all times.	1 2 3 4 5 N/A
12	The lancet gives indication of safety feature activation.	1 2 3 4 5 N/A
13	The lancet provides audible feedback that the safety feature has been activated.	1 2 3 4 5 N/A
14	The lancet provides visual feedback that the safety feature has been activated.	1 2 3 4 5 N/A
15	The lancet has an undefeatable safety feature that provides permanent coverage of the sharp.	1 2 3 4 5 N/A
16	The safety lancet operates reliably.	1 2 3 4 5 N/A
17	The design of the product suggests proper use.	1 2 3 4 5 N/A

Of the above questions, which three are the most important to your safety when using this product?

Are there other questions which you feel should be asked regarding the safety features of this product?

© 2005 International Sharps Injury Prevention Society – modeled after evaluation forms copyrighted by TDICT

SAFETY FEATURE EVALUATION FORM
SHARPS DISPOSAL CONTAINERS

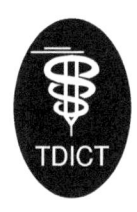

Date: _____ Department: _____ Occupation: _____

Product: _____ Number of times used: _____

Please **circle** the most appropriate answer for each question. Not applicable (N/A) may be used if the question does not apply to this particular product.

---

agree............disagree

1. The container's shape, its markings, or its color, imply danger..................................1 2 3 4 5 N/A
2. The implied warning of danger can be seen from the angle at which people commonly view it. (very short people, people in wheel chairs, children, etc.).......... 1 2 3 4 5 N/A
3. The implied warning can be universally understood by visitors, children, and patients. .... 1 2 3 4 5 N/A
4. The container's purpose is self-explanatory and easily understood by a worker who may be pressed for time or unfamiliar with the hospital setting......................... 1 2 3 4 5 N/A
5. The container can accept sharps from any direction desired.................................. 1 2 3 4 5 N/A
6. The container can accept all sizes and shapes of sharps....................................... 1 2 3 4 5 N/A
7. The container allows single handed operation. (Only the hand holding the sharp should be near the container opening.)... 1 2 3 4 5 N/A
8. It is difficult to reach in and remove a sharp. .... 1 2 3 4 5 N/A
9. Sharps can go into the container without getting caught on the opening................ 1 2 3 4 5 N/A
10. Sharps can go into tthe container without getting caught on any molded shapes in the interior.. 1 2 3 4 5 N/A
11. The container is puncture resistant.. 1 2 3 4 5 N/A
12. When the container is dropped or turned upside down (even before it is permanently closed) sharps stay inside... 1 2 3 4 5 N/A
13. The user can determine easily, from various viewing angles, when the container is full.. 1 2 3 4 5 N/A
14. When the container is to be used free-standing (no mounting bracket), it is stable and unlikely to tip over.. 1 2 3 4 5 N/A
15. It is safe to close the container. (Sharps should not protrude into the path of hands attempting to close the container.)... 1 2 3 4 5 N/A
16. The container closes securely. (e.g. if the closure requires glue, it may not work if the surfaces are soiled or wet.)... 1 2 3 4 5 N/A
17. The product has handles which allow you to safely transport a full container... 1 2 3 4 5 N/A
18. The product **does not** require extensive training to operate correctly..................... 1 2 3 4 5 N/A

Of the above questions, which three are the most important to **your** safety when using this product?

Are there other questions which you feel should be asked regarding the safety/ utility of this product?

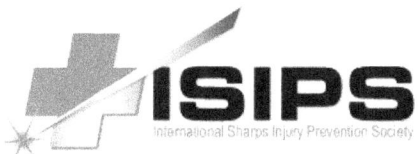

TUBES AND CONTAINERS EVALUATION FORM

Date: _____ Department: _____

Evaluator: _____ Product: _____ Number of times used: _____

Please **circle** the most appropriate answer for each question. Not applicable (N/A) may be used if the question does not apply to this particular product.

		Agree.........Disagree
1	The tube or container is made of plastic.	1 2 3 4 5 N/A
2	This device provides a better alternative to traditional product made out of glass.	1 2 3 4 5 N/A
3	This product is no more difficult to use than traditional winged needles and requires no additional time.	1 2 3 4 5 N/A
4	The product works well with a wide variety of hand sizes.	1 2 3 4 5 N/A
5	The product is easy to handle while wearing gloves.	1 2 3 4 5 N/A
6	The product can be used by either right or left handed clinicians.	1 2 3 4 5 N/A
7	The safety feature of the product does not cause interference with the procedure.	1 2 3 4 5 N/A
8	The user does not need extensive training for correct use of the product.	1 2 3 4 5 N/A
9	The product is suitable for a range of uses across a variety of patient populations.	1 2 3 4 5 N/A
10	The safety feature of the product is a passive feature; it requires no intervention on the part of the clinician to activate.	1 2 3 4 5 N/A
11	The user's hands are protected from a sharp at all times.	1 2 3 4 5 N/A
12	The product operates reliably.	1 2 3 4 5 N/A
13	The design of the product suggests proper use.	1 2 3 4 5 N/A
14	Use of the product requires you to use the safety feature.	1 2 3 4 5 N/A

Of the above questions, which three are the most important to your safety when using this product?

Are there other questions which you feel should be asked regarding the safety features of this product?

Conclusions: _____

_____

_____

SAFETY FEATURE EVALUATION FORM
VACUUM TUBE BLOOD COLLECTION SYSTEMS

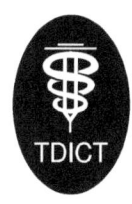

Date: _____ Department: _____ Occupation: _____

Product: _____ Number of times used: _____

Please **circle** the most appropriate answer for each question. Not applicable (N/A) may be used if the question does not apply to this particular product.

		agree............disagree
1.	The safety feature can be activated using a one-handed technique.........................	1 2 3 4 5 N/A
2.	The safety feature **does not** interfere with normal use of this product......................	1 2 3 4 5 N/A
3.	Use of this product requires you to use the safety feature..	1 2 3 4 5 N/A
4.	This product **does not** require more time to use than a non-safety device..............	1 2 3 4 5 N/A
5.	The safety feature works well with a wide variety of hand sizes............................	1 2 3 4 5 N/A
6.	The safety feature works with a butterfly..	1 2 3 4 5 N/A
7.	A clear and unmistakable change (either audible or visible) occurs when the safety feature is activated..	1 2 3 4 5 N/A
8.	The safety feature operates reliably..	1 2 3 4 5 N/A
9.	The exposed sharp is blunted or covered after use and prior to disposal................	1 2 3 4 5 N/A
10.	The inner vacuum tube needle (rubber sleeved needle) **does not** present a danger of exposure...	1 2 3 4 5 N/A
11.	The **product does** not need extensive training to be operated correctly..................	1 2 3 4 5 N/A

Of the above questions, which three are the most important to **your** safety when using this product?

Are there other questions which you feel should be asked regarding the safety/ utility of this product?

Medical Devices for Biomedical Safety

Amniocentesis Trays

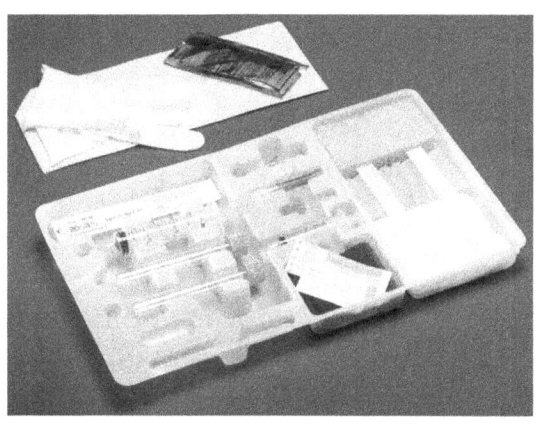

Curity™ Amniocentesis Tray

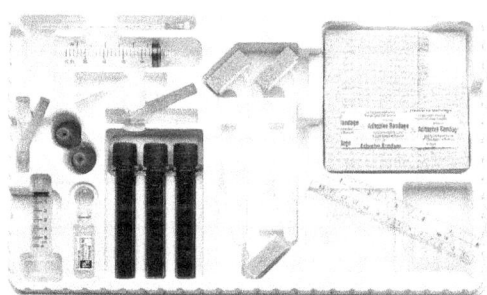

Safe-T-Amnio™ Tray

Curity™ Amniocentesis Tray

Device Description:
The Curity Amniocentesis Tray is a high-quality disposable tray that contains all the components necessary for the aspiration of amniotic fluid. Features a 20ga x 3 1/2" Amniocentesis Needle.

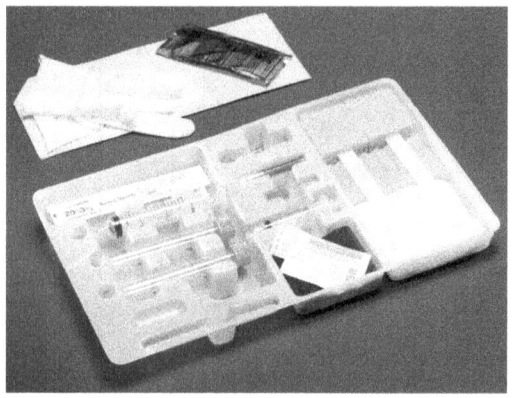

Advantages:
Each high quality procedure tray features Monoject™ Magellan safety needles and a retractable scalpel.

Safety Features and Benefits:
Safety Needle prevents accidental needlesticks.

Mechanics:
Each procedure tray comes with all components necessary to complete the procedure and features the Monoject Magellan Needle.

FDA Status:	Approved
Sizes Available:	20ga x 3 1/2"
Product Website:	www.kendallhq.com
Brochure Download:	
Instructional Website:	
Instructional Video:	
Contact for Samples:	
Contact for Purchase:	Contact your Local Sales Rep @1-800-962-9888. Product can also be obtained via your dealer of choice
Availability:	Now available
Manufacturer:	Kendall Healthcare 15 Hampshire Street Mansfield, MA 02762 USA 508-261-8637 paula.girvan@tycohealthcare.com

Amniocentesis Tray

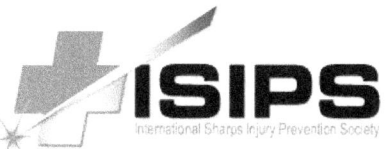

SAFETY SCALPEL EVALUATION FORM

Date: _____ Department: _____

Evaluator: _____ Product: _____ Number of times used: _____

Please **circle** the most appropriate answer for each question. Not applicable (N/A) may be used if the question does not apply to this particular product.

		Agree.........Disagree
1	The safety feature of the scalpel can be activated using a one-handed technique.	1 2 3 4 5 N/A
2	The safety feature does not obstruct vision of the tip of the scalpel blade.	1 2 3 4 5 N/A
3	Use of this product requires you to use the safety feature.	1 2 3 4 5 N/A
4	This product does not require more time to use than a non-safety device.	1 2 3 4 5 N/A
5	The safety feature works well with a wide variety of hand sizes.	1 2 3 4 5 N/A
6	The device is easy to handle while wearing gloves.	1 2 3 4 5 N/A
7	This device provides a better alternative to traditional scalpels.	1 2 3 4 5 N/A
8	There is a clear and unmistakable change (audible or visible) that occurs when the safety feature is activated.	1 2 3 4 5 N/A
9	The safety feature operates reliably.	1 2 3 4 5 N/A
10	The safety feature has three positions: blade exposed, blade covered, blade permanently locked.	1 2 3 4 5 N/A
11	After being placed in the permanently locked position the safety feature cannot be undone.	1 2 3 4 5 N/A
12	This safety scalpel is no more difficult to use than non-safety scalpels.	1 2 3 4 5 N/A
13	The user does not need extensive training for correct use of the product.	1 2 3 4 5 N/A
14	The design of the product suggests proper use.	1 2 3 4 5 N/A
15	It is not easy to skip a crucial step in proper use of the device.	1 2 3 4 5 N/A
16	The product can be easily used in the right hand.	1 2 3 4 5 N/A
17	The product can be easily used in the left hand.	1 2 3 4 5 N/A
18	The product can be easily used in either hand.	1 2 3 4 5 N/A
19	The use of the product does not require passing scalpel with the blade exposed.	1 2 3 4 5 N/A
20	The handle is similar in size and weight to standard scalpel.	1 2 3 4 5 N/A
21	The scalpel handle has grips for stable handling.	1 2 3 4 5 N/A

Of the above questions, which three are the most important to your safety when using this product?

Are there other questions which you feel should be asked regarding the safety features of this product?

Safe-T-Amnio™ Tray

Device Description:
Single-use, sterile Safe-T-Amnio™ trays and standard amniocentesis trays are available in a variety of configurations for your procedural needs.

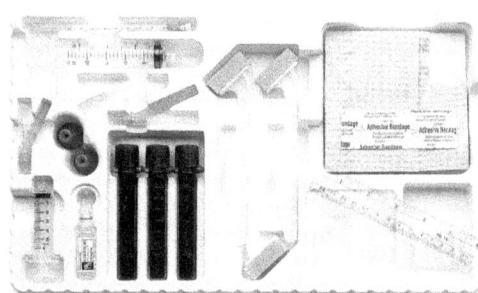

Safe-T-Amnio™ Tray

Advantages:
Match-ground needles help eliminate tissue coring.Ultra sharp, long bevel tip geometry facilitates easy insertion & reduces pain. Cm depth markings assist in precise needle positioning. Ultra-clear hubs w/magnification window & side view channels provide 360° visibility. Blue tint increases visualization & helps reduce glare. Non-slip wings facilitate positive handling during insertion.

Safety Features and Benefits:
The Portex® Brand Needle-Pro® Hypodermic System is a combination of a hypodermic needle system and a hinged protective sheath that covers the contaminated needle upon activation using a simple, one-handed technique. The Portex® Brand Point-Lok® Freestanding Protection Device is designed to lock onto and contain a single contaminated needle. The Point-Lok device is used with instruments such as spinal needles for which integrated ESIP technology cannot feasibly be used.

Mechanics:
Amniocentesis is performed by following standard amniocentesis procedure. Safety devices (Portex Needle-Pro and Portex Point Lok) are included in the tray to help prevent needlesticks.

FDA Status:	Approved
Sizes Available:	4545AS Safe-T-Amnio™ tray with 20G x 31⁄2˝ (8.9cm) spinal needle
Product Website:	http://www.cardinal.com/mps/brands/specialprocedures/safettrays.asp
Brochure Download:	http://www.cardinal.com/mps/brands/specialprocedures/safettray.pdf
Instructional Website:	N/A
Instructional Video:	N/A
Contact for Samples:	
Contact for Purchase:	To place an order, contact your Cardinal Health sales representative or call 800-964-5227.
Availability:	Now available
Manufacturer:	Cardinal Health 1430 Waukegan Rd. KB-B3 McGaw Park, IL 60085 USA 847-578-6457 www,cardinal.com linda.scott@cardinal.com

CardinalHealth

Amniocentesis Tray

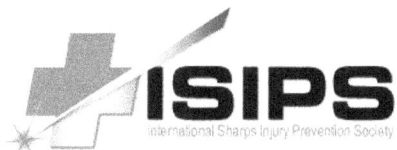

SAFETY SCALPEL EVALUATION FORM

Date: _____ Department: _____

Evaluator: _____ Product: _____ Number of times used: _____

Please **circle** the most appropriate answer for each question. Not applicable (N/A) may be used if the question does not apply to this particular product.

		Agree.........Disagree
1	The safety feature of the scalpel can be activated using a one-handed technique.	1 2 3 4 5 N/A
2	The safety feature does not obstruct vision of the tip of the scalpel blade.	1 2 3 4 5 N/A
3	Use of this product requires you to use the safety feature.	1 2 3 4 5 N/A
4	This product does not require more time to use than a non-safety device.	1 2 3 4 5 N/A
5	The safety feature works well with a wide variety of hand sizes.	1 2 3 4 5 N/A
6	The device is easy to handle while wearing gloves.	1 2 3 4 5 N/A
7	This device provides a better alternative to traditional scalpels.	1 2 3 4 5 N/A
8	There is a clear and unmistakable change (audible or visible) that occurs when the safety feature is activated.	1 2 3 4 5 N/A
9	The safety feature operates reliably.	1 2 3 4 5 N/A
10	The safety feature has three positions: blade exposed, blade covered, blade permanently locked.	1 2 3 4 5 N/A
11	After being placed in the permanently locked position the safety feature cannot be undone.	1 2 3 4 5 N/A
12	This safety scalpel is no more difficult to use than non-safety scalpels.	1 2 3 4 5 N/A
13	The user does not need extensive training for correct use of the product.	1 2 3 4 5 N/A
14	The design of the product suggests proper use.	1 2 3 4 5 N/A
15	It is not easy to skip a crucial step in proper use of the device.	1 2 3 4 5 N/A
16	The product can be easily used in the right hand.	1 2 3 4 5 N/A
17	The product can be easily used in the left hand.	1 2 3 4 5 N/A
18	The product can be easily used in either hand.	1 2 3 4 5 N/A
19	The use of the product does not require passing scalpel with the blade exposed.	1 2 3 4 5 N/A
20	The handle is similar in size and weight to standard scalpel.	1 2 3 4 5 N/A
21	The scalpel handle has grips for stable handling.	1 2 3 4 5 N/A

Of the above questions, which three are the most important to your safety when using this product?

Are there other questions which you feel should be asked regarding the safety features of this product?

Medical Devices for Biomedical Safety

Blood Collection Equipment

Defender Safety Needle Holder

DonorCare® Needle Guard

Haemo-Diff Blood Smear

Maximus Blood Collection and Transfer Devices

Microvette® Capillary Blood Collection System

Monoject Angel Wing Safety Blood Collection

Needle Protector

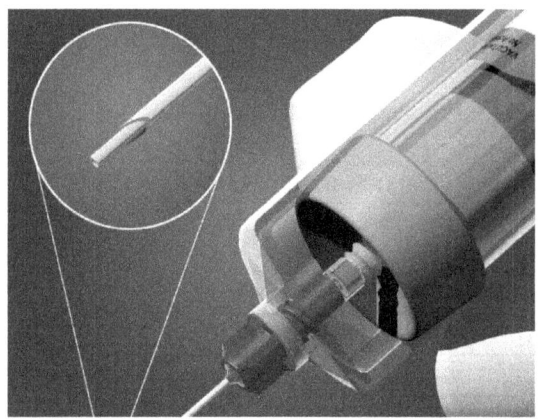

Punctur-Guard

Blood Collection Needles

Punctur-Guard Winged Set for Blood Collection

S-Monovette® Blood Collection System

Saf-T Holder® Devices

Saf-T Wing® Blood Collection Set

Samploc® Sampling Kit

Continued Next Page

VACUETTE® QUICKSHIELD Safety Tube Holder

VACUETTE® Safety Blood Collection Set

VanishPoint® Blood Collection System

Venipuncture Needle-Pro® Device

Capiject ® capillary blood collection tubes

Device Description:
Capiject plastic tubes are used for capillary blood collection, when blood is being collected by gravity flow.

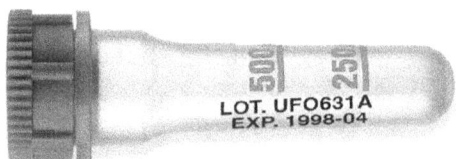

Capiject color coded tubes

Advantages:
Capiject tubes have an extra-wide collection lip for enhanced specimen flow, and single piece design, tapered design for easy collection and handling. Capiject tubes are latex free and certified for lead testing.

Safety Features and Benefits:
Capiject tubes are plastic and have no extra accessory pieces that will require disposal prior to processing.

Mechanics:
Capiject tubes are have built-in collection lip to enhance specimen flow. The tubes nest in the color coded caps, allowing tubes to stand alone.

FDA Status:	Approved
Sizes Available:	Full range of collection tubes for serum, plasma, and whole blood determinations.
Product Website:	www.terumomedical.com
Brochure Download:	www.terumomedical.com
Instructional Website:	www.terumomedical.com
Instructional Video:	
Contact for Samples:	
Contact for Purchase:	Product can be ordered directly from Terumo or through most healthcare distributors.
Availability:	Now available
Manufacturer:	Terumo Medical 2101 Cottontail Lane Somerset,, NJ 08873 USA 732-302-4911 www.terumomedical.com safety.sharps@terumomedical.com

Blood Collection Equipment

SAFETY FEATURE EVALUATION FORM
I.V. ACCESS DEVICES

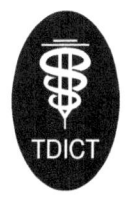

Date: _____ Department: _____ Occupation: _____

Product: _____ Number of times used: _____

Please **circle** the most appropriate answer for each question. Not applicable (N/A) may be used if the question does not apply to this particular product.

agree............disagree

1. The safety feature can be activated using a one-handed technique......................... 1 2 3 4 5 N/A
2. The safety feature **does not** interfere with normal use of this product..................... 1 2 3 4 5 N/A
3. Use of this product requires you to use the safety feature...................................... 1 2 3 4 5 N/A
4. This product **does not** require more time to use than a non-safety device.............. 1 2 3 4 5 N/A
5. The safety feature works well with a wide variety of hand sizes............................ 1 2 3 4 5 N/A
6. The device allows for rapid visualization of flashback in the catheter or chamber... 1 2 3 4 5 N/A
7. Use of this product **does not** increase the number of sticks to the patient..............1 2 3 4 5 N/A
8. The product stops the flow of blood after the needle is removed from the catheter (or after the butterfly is inserted) and just prior to line connections or hep-lock capping.. 1 2 3 4 5 N/A
9. A clear and unmistakable change (either audible or visible) occurs when the safety feature is activated............................... .... 1 2 3 4 5 N/A
10. The safety feature operates reliably.. 1 2 3 4 5 N/A
11. The exposed sharp is blunted or covered after use and prior to disposal.............. 1 2 3 4 5 N/A
12. The product **does not** need extensive training to be operated correctly................. 1 2 3 4 5 N/A

Of the above questions, which three are the most important to **your** safety when using this product?

Are there other questions which you feel should be asked regarding the safety/ utility of this product?

Defender Safety Needle Holder

Device Description:
Defender Safety Phlebotomy Needle Holder is designed to comply with OSHA's Bloodborne Pathogen Standards while providing clinicians easy activation. Defender provides one-handed activation and simultaneous front and back-end needle protection.

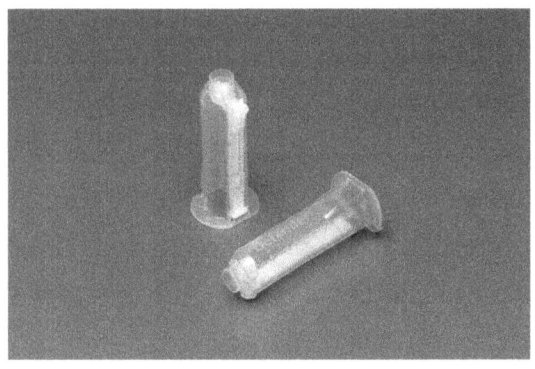

Advantages:
Complete needle retraction, one-handed activation, integral safety shield, single-use design, back-end protection, easy/intuitive activation.

Safety Features and Benefits:
Complies with OSHA Bloodborne Pathogens Standard for Engineering controls, provides barrier from needle, hands remain behind needle, integral safety mechanism.

FDA Status:	Approved
Sizes Available:	1
Product Website:	www.tycohealthcare.com
Brochure Download:	www.tycohealthcare.com
Instructional Website:	www.tycohealthcare.com
Instructional Video:	www.tycohealthcare.com
Contact for Samples:	
Contact for Purchase:	Contact Kendall SharpSafety Representative.
Availability:	Now available
Manufacturer:	Tyco Healthcare/ Kendall 15 Hampshire Street Mansfield, MA 02048 USA 508-261-8456 www.kendallhq.com Tony.Sacchetti@tycohealthcare.com

Blood Collection Equipment

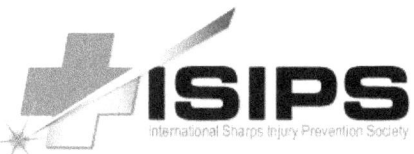

TUBES AND CONTAINERS EVALUATION FORM

Date: _____ Department: _____

Evaluator: _____ Product: _____ Number of times used: _____

Please **circle** the most appropriate answer for each question. Not applicable (N/A) may be used if the question does not apply to this particular product.

		Agree.........Disagree
1	The tube or container is made of plastic.	1 2 3 4 5 N/A
2	This device provides a better alternative to traditional product made out of glass.	1 2 3 4 5 N/A
3	This product is no more difficult to use than traditional winged needles and requires no additional time.	1 2 3 4 5 N/A
4	The product works well with a wide variety of hand sizes.	1 2 3 4 5 N/A
5	The product is easy to handle while wearing gloves.	1 2 3 4 5 N/A
6	The product can be used by either right or left handed clinicians.	1 2 3 4 5 N/A
7	The safety feature of the product does not cause interference with the procedure.	1 2 3 4 5 N/A
8	The user does not need extensive training for correct use of the product.	1 2 3 4 5 N/A
9	The product is suitable for a range of uses across a variety of patient populations.	1 2 3 4 5 N/A
10	The safety feature of the product is a passive feature; it requires no intervention on the part of the clinician to activate.	1 2 3 4 5 N/A
11	The user's hands are protected from a sharp at all times.	1 2 3 4 5 N/A
12	The product operates reliably.	1 2 3 4 5 N/A
13	The design of the product suggests proper use.	1 2 3 4 5 N/A
14	Use of the product requires you to use the safety feature.	1 2 3 4 5 N/A

Of the above questions, which three are the most important to your safety when using this product?

Are there other questions which you feel should be asked regarding the safety features of this product?

Conclusions: _____

_____

_____

_____

Haemo-Diff Blood Smear

Device Description:
Sarstedt's Haemo-Diff Blood Smear is designed specifically to work with the S-Monovette® Blood Collection System. The unique device creates a blood droplet directly from the closed S-Monovette® tube and smears this droplet onto the slide. This double function minimizes exposure to bloodborne pathogens and eliminates the need for additional products.

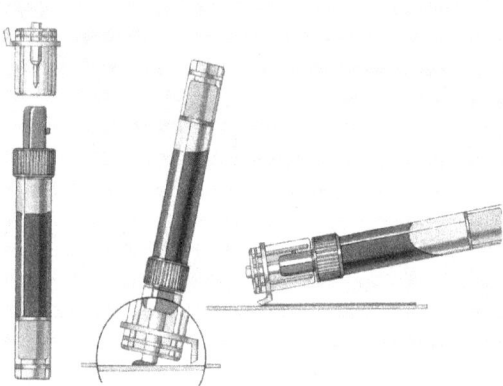

Advantages:
Place the Haemo-Diff vertically onto the S-Monovette®, piercing the membrane. Place the Haemo-Diff in a sloping position onto the slide to dispense a droplet of blood. Move the Haemo-Diff toward the droplet as usual to create a smear.

Safety Features and Benefits:
The Sarstedt Haemo-Diff minimizes exposure to bloodborne pathogens because opening of the tube is no longer required during slide preparation. The dual-function device also saves time and material costs.

FDA Status:	Listed
Sizes Available:	One size fits all S-Monovette® tubes
Product Website:	www.sarstedt.com/php/produktfamilie-darstellung.php?familie_id=112&seite=1
Brochure Download:	www.sarstedt.com/php/prospektanforderung.php?selected_gruppe_id=11
Instructional Website:	www.sarstedt.com/php/produktfamilie-darstellung.php?familie_id=112&seite=1
Instructional Video:	
Contact for Samples:	
Contact for Purchase:	(800) 257-5101; sarstedt@bellsouth.net; www.sarstedt.com/php/email.php
Availability:	Now available
Manufacturer:	Sarstedt, Inc. 1025 St. James Church Road P.O. Box 468 Newton, NC 28658 USA 800-257-5101 www.sarstedt.com sarstedt@bellsouth.net

Blood Collection Equipment

SARSTEDT

SAFETY FEATURE EVALUATION FORM
VACUUM TUBE BLOOD COLLECTION SYSTEMS

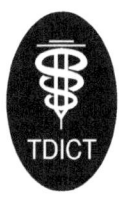

Date: _____ Department: _____ Occupation: _____

Product: _____ Number of times used: _____

Please **circle** the most appropriate answer for each question. Not applicable (N/A) may be used if the question does not apply to this particular product.

		agree..........disagree
1.	The safety feature can be activated using a one-handed technique........................	1 2 3 4 5 N/A
2.	The safety feature **does not** interfere with normal use of this product.....................	1 2 3 4 5 N/A
3.	Use of this product requires you to use the safety feature....................................	1 2 3 4 5 N/A
4.	This product **does not** require more time to use than a non-safety device..............	1 2 3 4 5 N/A
5.	The safety feature works well with a wide variety of hand sizes............................	1 2 3 4 5 N/A
6.	The safety feature works with a butterfly..	1 2 3 4 5 N/A
7.	A clear and unmistakable change (either audible or visible) occurs when the safety feature is activated..	1 2 3 4 5 N/A
8.	The safety feature operates reliably...	1 2 3 4 5 N/A
9.	The exposed sharp is blunted or covered after use and prior to disposal...............	1 2 3 4 5 N/A
10.	The inner vacuum tube needle (rubber sleeved needle) **does not** present a danger of exposure..	1 2 3 4 5 N/A
11.	The **product does** not need extensive training to be operated correctly.................	1 2 3 4 5 N/A

Of the above questions, which three are the most important to **your** safety when using this product?

Are there other questions which you feel should be asked regarding the safety/ utility of this product?

DonorCare® Needle Guard

Device Description:
The DonorCare® Needle Guard provides immediate shielding of the blood donation needle on withdrawal from the vein. DonorCare® has a two-stage engagement mechanism. The Engaged position stabilizes the needle hub while allowing for needle adjustment during collection. The Locked position shields and locks the needle preventing any possibility of needle stick injury.

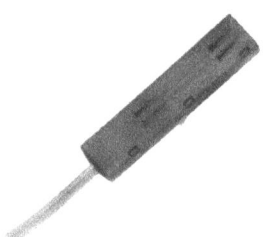

DonorCare® Needle Guard

Advantages:
Advantages include compatibility for use with current blood collection sets produced by all major manufacturers, an inexpensive cost, and ease of use and implementation. DonorCare® reduces the risk of donor/patient injury and trauma by stabilizing the needle hub, and it improves donor/patient comfort on withdrawal of the needle.

Safety Features and Benefits:
Safety benefits include the facilitation of a safe, fast needle withdrawal in emergency situations and ultimately a reduced risk of needle stick injury from both the donor/patient and sampling needles. Use of this needle guard also improves safety for subsequent procedures, including stripping, transportation and segmenting.

FDA Status:	Approved
Sizes Available:	Small Channel and Large Channel sizes available
Product Website:	www.itlcorporation.com
Brochure Download:	www.itlcorporation.com
Instructional Website:	www.itlcorporation.com
Instructional Video:	www.itlcorporation.com
Contact for Samples:	
Contact for Purchase:	Purchase orders can be placed by fax at (703) 435-6717 or by email at sales@itlus.com
Availability:	Now available
Manufacturer:	ITL Corporation 1175 Herndon Parkway Suite 350 Herndon, VA 20170 USA 703-435-6700 www.itlcorporation.com sales@itlus.com

Blood Collection Equipment

ITL CORPORATION

Safety Feature Evaluation Form
VACUUM TUBE BLOOD COLLECTION SYSTEMS

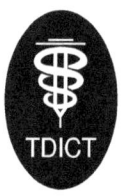

Date: _____ Department: _____ Occupation: _____

Product: _____ Number of times used: _____

Please **circle** the most appropriate answer for each question. Not applicable (N/A) may be used if the question does not apply to this particular product.

agree............disagree

1. The safety feature can be activated using a one-handed technique........................ 1 2 3 4 5 N/A
2. The safety feature **does not** interfere with normal use of this product......................1 2 3 4 5 N/A
3. Use of this product requires you to use the safety feature...................................... 1 2 3 4 5 N/A
4. This product **does not** require more time to use than a non-safety device.............. 1 2 3 4 5 N/A
5. The safety feature works well with a wide variety of hand sizes............................ 1 2 3 4 5 N/A
6. The safety feature works with a butterfly... 1 2 3 4 5 N/A
7. A clear and unmistakable change (either audible or visible) occurs when the
    safety feature is activated.. 1 2 3 4 5 N/A
8. The safety feature operates reliably.. 1 2 3 4 5 N/A
9. The exposed sharp is blunted or covered after use and prior to disposal................ 1 2 3 4 5 N/A
10. The inner vacuum tube needle (rubber sleeved needle) **does not** present a
    danger of exposure.. 1 2 3 4 5 N/A
11. The **product does** not need extensive training to be operated correctly.................1 2 3 4 5 N/A

Of the above questions, which three are the most important to **your** safety when using this product?

Are there other questions which you feel should be asked regarding the safety/ utility of this product?

Maximus Blood Collection and Transfer Devices

Device Description:

When partnered with the MaxPlus Needleless Access Device, both the Maximus Blood Collection Device with Luer Lock and the Maximus Blood Transfer Device allow quick and easy blood collection without exposure to a needle. Both of these products from Maximus Medical, a Quality Brand of Medegen, will not only make the process of collecting blood quicker and easier but more importantly safer.

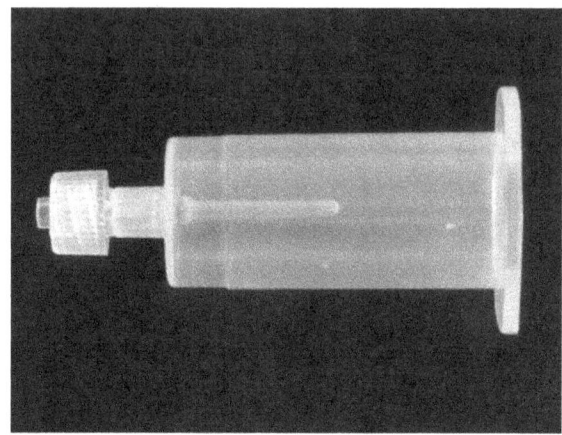

Advantages:

The Maximus Blood Collection Device provides a secure connection to the MaxPlus because of its luer lock. With its secure connection, the user need not worry about inadvertent disconnect which can occur with luer slip connections. The Blood Transfer Device gives the user the choice of using a syringe to draw the blood safely from the MaxPlus and then securely transferring it to a vacuum tube.

Safety Features and Benefits:

The Maximus Blood Transfer Device and Collection devices allow the user no exposure to a needle and no exposure to the blood that is being transferred. The two devices were designed with the users safety in mind. The Maximus Blood Collection and Blood Transfer Device give the user unsurpassed safety and ease of use.

FDA Status:	Approved
Sizes Available:	
Product Website:	www.medegen.com
Brochure Download:	
Instructional Website:	
Instructional Video:	
Contact for Samples:	Visit the Medical Safety Book.com Sample Procurement Center
Contact for Purchase:	
Availability:	Now available
Manufacturer:	Medegen 390 Wanamaker Ave Ontario, CA 91761 USA 909-390-9080 www.medegen.com janice.tarwater@medegen.com

Blood Collection Equipment

SAFETY FEATURE EVALUATION FORM
I.V. ACCESS DEVICES

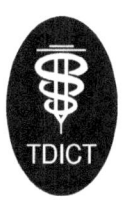

Date: _____ Department: _____ Occupation: _____

Product: _____ Number of times used: _____

Please **circle** the most appropriate answer for each question. Not applicable (N/A) may be used if the question does not apply to this particular product.

agree...........disagree

1. The safety feature can be activated using a one-handed technique........................ 1 2 3 4 5 N/A
2. The safety feature **does not** interfere with normal use of this product.................... 1 2 3 4 5 N/A
3. Use of this product requires you to use the safety feature...................................... 1 2 3 4 5 N/A
4. This product **does not** require more time to use than a non-safety device.............. 1 2 3 4 5 N/A
5. The safety feature works well with a wide variety of hand sizes............................ 1 2 3 4 5 N/A
6. The device allows for rapid visualization of flashback in the catheter or chamber... 1 2 3 4 5 N/A
7. Use of this product **does not** increase the number of sticks to the patient...............1 2 3 4 5 N/A
8. The product stops the flow of blood after the needle is removed from the catheter (or after the butterfly is inserted) and just prior to line connections or hep-lock capping.. 1 2 3 4 5 N/A
9. A clear and unmistakable change (either audible or visible) occurs when the safety feature is activated.. 1 2 3 4 5 N/A
10. The safety feature operates reliably... 1 2 3 4 5 N/A
11. The exposed sharp is blunted or covered after use and prior to disposal.............. 1 2 3 4 5 N/A
12. The product **does not** need extensive training to be operated correctly.................. 1 2 3 4 5 N/A

Of the above questions, which three are the most important to **your** safety when using this product?

Are there other questions which you feel should be asked regarding the safety/ utility of this product?

Microvette® Capillary Blood Collection System

Device Description:

Sarstedt's Microvette® Capillary Blood Collection System is a safe and reliable system for the collection of 100 to 500µl. Microvette® 100 and 200, for 100 and 200µl volumes respectively, are designed with pre-assembled capillaries. Microvette® 300 and 500, for 300 and 500µl volumes respectively, are designed with special rims for the gravity flow principle of collection. Both versions have twist caps to minimize aerosols and are available in a full range of additives.

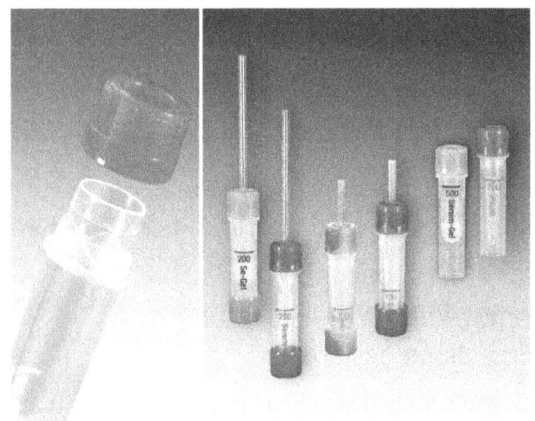

Mechanics of the Device:

100 and 200µl: Collect blood until the assembled capillary is filled. Turn the tube upright to allow the blood to flow into the Microvette® tube. Turn the cap to remove and discard the pre-assembled capillary as one unit. Remove the cap from the base and seal the Microvette®. 300 and 500µl: Remove the twist cap and attach it to the base of the Microvette®. Collect blood using any part of the collection rim. Remove the cap from the base and seal the Microvette®.

Safety Features and Benefits:

Sarstedt's Microvette® Capillary Blood Collection System features an easy-to-use twist cap to reduce exposure to bloodborne pathogens via aerosols. Smooth tube interiors prevent sample hold-up, allowing optimal sample mixing and recovery.

FDA Status:	Listed
Sizes Available:	Full range of volumes and additives
Product Website:	www.sarstedt.com/php/produktfamilie-darstellung.php?familie_id=114&seite=0
Brochure Download:	www.sarstedt.com/php/prospektanforderung.php?selected_gruppe_id=11
Instructional Website:	www.sarstedt.com/php/produktfamilie-darstellung.php?familie_id=114&seite=0
Instructional Video:	
Contact for Samples:	Visit the Medical Safety Book.com Sample Procurement Center
Contact for Purchase:	(800) 257-5101; sarstedt@bellsouth.net; www.sarstedt.com/php/email.php
Availability:	Now available
Manufacturer:	Sarstedt, Inc. 1025 St. James Church Road P.O. Box 468 Newton, NC 28658 USA 800-257-5101 www.sarstedt.com sarstedt@bellsouth.net

SARSTEDT

Blood Collection Equipment

SAFETY FEATURE EVALUATION FORM
VACUUM TUBE BLOOD COLLECTION SYSTEMS

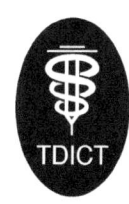

Date: _____ Department: _____ Occupation: _____

Product: _____ Number of times used: _____

Please **circle** the most appropriate answer for each question. Not applicable (N/A) may be used if the question does not apply to this particular product.

agree............disagree

1. The safety feature can be activated using a one-handed technique........................ 1 2 3 4 5 N/A
2. The safety feature **does not** interfere with normal use of this product.....................1 2 3 4 5 N/A
3. Use of this product requires you to use the safety feature...................................... 1 2 3 4 5 N/A
4. This product **does not** require more time to use than a non-safety device.............. 1 2 3 4 5 N/A
5. The safety feature works well with a wide variety of hand sizes............................. 1 2 3 4 5 N/A
6. The safety feature works with a butterfly... 1 2 3 4 5 N/A
7. A clear and unmistakable change (either audible or visible) occurs when the safety feature is activated... 1 2 3 4 5 N/A
8. The safety feature operates reliably... 1 2 3 4 5 N/A
9. The exposed sharp is blunted or covered after use and prior to disposal................ 1 2 3 4 5 N/A
10. The inner vacuum tube needle (rubber sleeved needle) **does not** present a danger of exposure... 1 2 3 4 5 N/A
11. The **product does** not need extensive training to be operated correctly..................1 2 3 4 5 N/A

Of the above questions, which three are the most important to **your** safety when using this product?

Are there other questions which you feel should be asked regarding the safety/ utility of this product?

Microvette® Capillary Blood Collection System

Device Description:
Sarstedt's Microvette® Capillary Blood Collection System is a safe and reliable system for the collection of 100 to 500µl. Microvette® 100 and 200, for 100 and 200µl volumes respectively, are designed with pre-assembled capillaries. Microvette® 300 and 500, for 300 and 500µl volumes respectively, are designed with special rims for the gravity flow principle of collection. Both versions have twist caps to minimize aerosols and are available in a full range of additives.

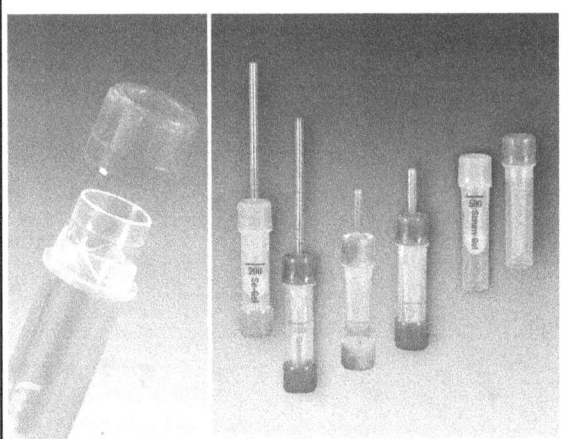

Advantages:
100 and 200µl: Collect blood until the assembled capillary is filled. Turn the tube upright to allow the blood to flow into the Microvette® tube. Turn the cap to remove and discard the pre-assembled capillary as one unit. Remove the cap from the base and seal the Microvette®. 300 and 500µl: Remove the twist cap and attach it to the base of the Microvette®. Collect blood using any part of the collection rim. Remove the cap from the base and seal the Microvette®.

Safety Features and Benefits:
Sarstedt's Microvette® Capillary Blood Collection System features an easy-to-use twist cap to reduce exposure to bloodborne pathogens via aerosols. Smooth tube interiors prevent sample hold-up, allowing optimal sample mixing and recovery.

FDA Status:	Listed
Sizes Available:	Full range of volumes and additives
Product Website:	www.sarstedt.com/php/produktfamilie-darstellung.php?familie_id=114&seite=0
Brochure Download:	www.sarstedt.com/php/prospektanforderung.php?selected_gruppe_id=11
Instructional Website:	www.sarstedt.com/php/produktfamilie-darstellung.php?familie_id=114&seite=0
Instructional Video:	
Contact for Samples:	
Contact for Purchase:	(800) 257-5101; sarstedt@bellsouth.net; www.sarstedt.com/php/email.php
Availability:	Now available
Manufacturer:	Sarstedt, Inc. 1025 St. James Church Road P.O. Box 468 Newton, NC 28658 USA 800-257-5101 www.sarstedt.com sarstedt@bellsouth.net

SARSTEDT

Blood Collection Equipment

SAFETY FEATURE EVALUATION FORM
VACUUM TUBE BLOOD COLLECTION SYSTEMS

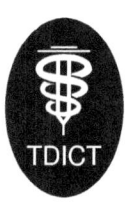

Date: _____ Department: _____ Occupation: _____

Product: _____ Number of times used: _____

Please **circle** the most appropriate answer for each question. Not applicable (N/A) may be used if the question does not apply to this particular product.

agree............disagree

1. The safety feature can be activated using a one-handed technique........................ 1 2 3 4 5 N/A
2. The safety feature **does not** interfere with normal use of this product...................... 1 2 3 4 5 N/A
3. Use of this product requires you to use the safety feature...................................... 1 2 3 4 5 N/A
4. This product **does not** require more time to use than a non-safety device.............. 1 2 3 4 5 N/A
5. The safety feature works well with a wide variety of hand sizes............................. 1 2 3 4 5 N/A
6. The safety feature works with a butterfly.. 1 2 3 4 5 N/A
7. A clear and unmistakable change (either audible or visible) occurs when the
   safety feature is activated... 1 2 3 4 5 N/A
8. The safety feature operates reliably.. 1 2 3 4 5 N/A
9. The exposed sharp is blunted or covered after use and prior to disposal................ 1 2 3 4 5 N/A
10. The inner vacuum tube needle (rubber sleeved needle) **does not** present a
    danger of exposure.. 1 2 3 4 5 N/A
11. The **product does** not need extensive training to be operated correctly................. 1 2 3 4 5 N/A

Of the above questions, which three are the most important to **your** safety when using this product?

Are there other questions which you feel should be asked regarding the safety/ utility of this product?

Training for Development of Innovative Control Technology Project

Monoject Angel Wing Safety Blood Collection

Device Description:

Kendall's Angel Wing Safety Needle System provides clinicians with a one-handed method of blood collection to effectively help protect against accidental needlesticks.

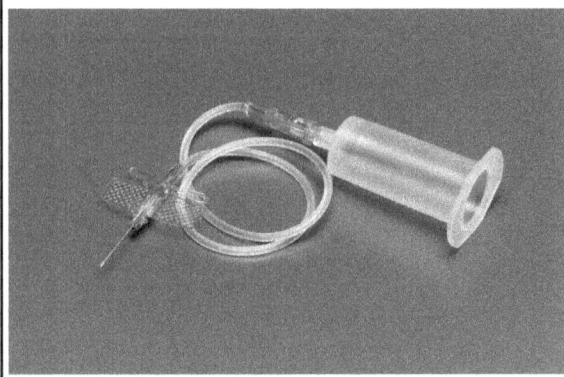

Advantages:

One-handed technique, textured wings, soft flexible tubing, four needle gauges available, available with or without multi-luer adapter or blood tube holder.

Safety Features and Benefits:

Complies with OSHA Bloodborne Pathogen Standard for Engineering Controls. One-handed protection against accidental needlesticks.

FDA Status:	Approved
Sizes Available:	19-25 gauge 3/4
Product Website:	www.tycohealthcare.com
Brochure Download:	www.tycohealthcare.com
Instructional Website:	www.tycohealthcare.com
Instructional Video:	www.tycohealthcare.com
Contact for Samples:	Visit the Medical Safety Book.com Sample Procurement Center
Contact for Purchase:	Contact Kendall SharpSafety Representative.
Availability:	Now available
Manufacturer:	Tyco Healthcare/ Kendall 15 Hampshire Street Mansfield, MA 02048 USA 508-261-8456 www.kendallhq.com Tony.Sacchetti@tycohealthcare.com

Blood Collection Equipment

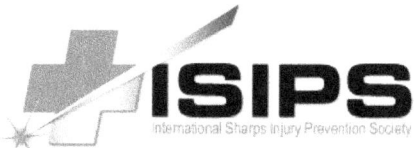

GENERIC SAFETY DEVICE EVALUATION FORM

Date: _____ Department:_____

Evaluator:_____ Product:_____ Number of times used:_____

Please **circle** the most appropriate answer for each question. Not applicable (N/A) may be used if the question does not apply to this particular product.

		Agree.........Disagree
1	The use of the device does not require extensive change in technique.	1 2 3 4 5 N/A
2	This device provides a better alternative to non-safety product.	1 2 3 4 5 N/A
3	This device is no more difficult to use than traditional non-safety product and requires no additional time.	1 2 3 4 5 N/A
4	The device works well with a wide variety of hand sizes.	1 2 3 4 5 N/A
5	The device is easy to handle while wearing gloves.	1 2 3 4 5 N/A
6	The device can be used by either right or left handed clinicians.	1 2 3 4 5 N/A
7	The safety feature of the device does not cause interference with the procedure.	1 2 3 4 5 N/A
8	The user does not need extensive training for correct use of the product.	1 2 3 4 5 N/A
9	The product is suitable for a range of uses across a variety of patient populations.	1 2 3 4 5 N/A
10	The safety feature of the product is a passive feature; it requires no intervention on the part of the clinician to activate.	1 2 3 4 5 N/A
11	The user's hands are protected from a sharp at all times.	1 2 3 4 5 N/A
12	The device gives indication of safety feature activation.	1 2 3 4 5 N/A
13	The device provides audible and visual feedback that the safety feature has been activated.	1 2 3 4 5 N/A
14	The device has an undefeatable safety feature that provides permanent coverage of the sharp.	1 2 3 4 5 N/A
15	The device operates reliably.	1 2 3 4 5 N/A
16	The design of the product suggests proper use.	1 2 3 4 5 N/A
17	Use of the product requires you to use the safety feature.	1 2 3 4 5 N/A
18	Use of the product removes a sharp thus removing potential for exposure to sharps injury and bloodborne pathogen exposure.	1 2 3 4 5 N/A

Of the above questions, which three are the most important to your safety when using this product?

Are there other questions which you feel should be asked regarding the safety features of this product?

Conclusions: _____

. _____

. _____

Needle Protector

Device Description:
Sarstedt's Needle Protector is designed specifically to work with the S-Monovette® blood collection needle. The device aids in protecting against needlestick injuries by completely enclosing the needle after it is removed from the vein. The Needle Protector fits all S-Monovette® needles.

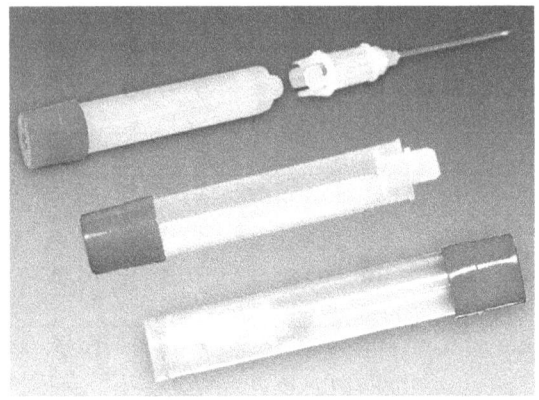

Mechanics of the Device:
Complete venous blood collection with the S-Monovette® Blood Collection System. Remove the last S-Monovette® tube, leaving the needle in the vein. Attach the Needle Protector to the needle with its locking pin mechanism. Remove the needle from the vein and draw it into the device. Lock the plunger into the base of the device and break it off. Invert the device and insert the plunger into the open end. Lock in the plunger by pressing firmly on the red cap.

Safety Features and Benefits:
The Sarstedt Needle Protector aids against needlestick injuries by completely enclosing the S-Monovette® needle after it is removed from the vein. The device fits all S-Monovette® needles, and its compact design minimizes disposal volume.

FDA Status:	Approved
Sizes Available:	One size fits all S-Monovette® needles
Product Website:	www.sarstedt.com/php/produktfamilie-darstellung.php?familie_id=117&seite=0
Brochure Download:	www.sarstedt.com/php/prospektanforderung.php?selected_gruppe_id=11
Instructional Website:	www.sarstedt.com/php/produktfamilie-darstellung.php?familie_id=117&seite=0
Instructional Video:	
Contact for Samples:	Visit the Medical Safety Book.com Sample Procurement Center
Contact for Purchase:	(800) 257-5101; sarstedt@bellsouth.net; www.sarstedt.com/php/email.php
Availability:	Now available
Manufacturer:	Sarstedt, Inc. 1025 St. James Church Road P.O. Box 468 Newton, NC 28658 USA 800-257-5101 www.sarstedt.com sarstedt@bellsouth.net

SARSTEDT

Blood Collection Equipment

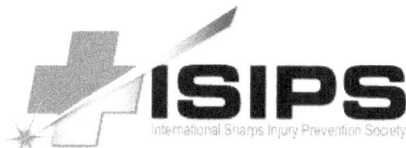

SAFETY WINGED NEEDLE EVALUATION FORM

Date: _____ Department: _____

Evaluator: _____ Product: _____ Number of times used: _____

Please **circle** the most appropriate answer for each question. Not applicable (N/A) may be used if the question does not apply to this particular product.

		Agree.........Disagree
1	The use of the Safety winged needle does not require extensive change in technique from the use of standard winged needles.	1 2 3 4 5 N/A
2	This device provides a better alternative to traditional winged needles.	1 2 3 4 5 N/A
3	This winged needle is no more difficult to use than traditional winged needles and requires no additional time.	1 2 3 4 5 N/A
4	The winged needle works well with a wide variety of hand sizes.	1 2 3 4 5 N/A
5	The winged needle is easy to handle while wearing gloves.	1 2 3 4 5 N/A
6	The winged needle can be used by either right or left handed clinicians.	1 2 3 4 5 N/A
7	The safety feature of the winged needle does not cause interference with the procedure.	1 2 3 4 5 N/A
8	The user does not need extensive training for correct use of the product.	1 2 3 4 5 N/A
9	The product is suitable for a range of uses across a variety of patient populations.	1 2 3 4 5 N/A
10	The safety feature of the product is a passive feature; it requires no intervention on the part of the clinician to activate.	1 2 3 4 5 N/A
11	The user's hands are protected from the sharp at all times.	1 2 3 4 5 N/A
12	The winged needle gives indication of safety feature activation.	1 2 3 4 5 N/A
13	The winged needle provides audible and visual feedback that the safety feature has been activated.	1 2 3 4 5 N/A
14	The winged needle has an undefeatable safety feature that provides permanent coverage of the sharp.	1 2 3 4 5 N/A
15	The winged needle operates reliably.	1 2 3 4 5 N/A
16	The design of the product suggests proper use.	1 2 3 4 5 N/A
17	The design of the safety winged needle allows it to be flush against skin without a high profile.	1 2 3 4 5 N/A
18	Use of the product requires you to use the safety feature.	1 2 3 4 5 N/A

Of the above questions, which three are the most important to your safety when using this product?

Are there other questions which you feel should be asked regarding the safety features of this product?

Conclusions: _____-

Punctur-Guard Blood Collection Needles

Device Description:
The Punctur-Guard blood collection needle is the only needle providing in-the-vein blunting technology. This offers the highest level of safety available as the device is rendered safe before leaving the patient's vein.

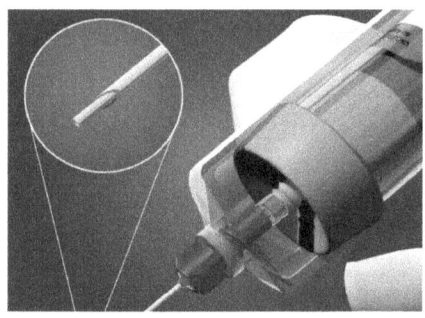

Punctur-Guard Blood Collection Needle

Advantages:
The primary advantage with the Punctur-Guard needle is the in-the-vien blunting technology. The Punctur-Guard eliminates the risk of sharps exposure during the first few critical seconds while withdrawing from the patient's vein. In a CDC stduy the Punctur-Guard reduced needlestick injury by 76%; the highest of any device studied. MMWR 1997, 46: 21-25.

Safety Features and Benefits:
In-the-vein blunting technology.

FDA Status:	Approved
Sizes Available:	21G, 22G
Product Website:	http://www.icumed.com/Punctureguard.asp
Brochure Download:	http://www.icumed.com/Punctureguard.asp
Instructional Website:	http://www.icumed.com/Punctureguard.asp
Instructional Video:	http://www.icumed.com/Punctureguard.asp
Contact for Samples:	Visit the Medical Safety Book.com Sample Procurement Center
Contact for Purchase:	Contact ICU Medical, Inc.
Availability:	Now available
Manufacturer:	ICU Medical, Inc. 951 Calle Amanecer San Clemente, CA 92673 USA 949-366-2183 www.icumed.com aburcar@icumed.com

Blood Collection Equipment

SAFETY FEATURE EVALUATION FORM
VACUUM TUBE BLOOD COLLECTION SYSTEMS

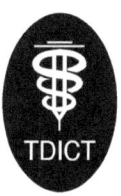

Date: _____ Department: _____ Occupation: _____

Product: _____ Number of times used: _____

Please **circle** the most appropriate answer for each question. Not applicable (N/A) may be used if the question does not apply to this particular product.

agree...........disagree

1. The safety feature can be activated using a one-handed technique........................ 1 2 3 4 5 N/A
2. The safety feature **does not** interfere with normal use of this product......................1 2 3 4 5 N/A
3. Use of this product requires you to use the safety feature...................................... 1 2 3 4 5 N/A
4. This product **does not** require more time to use than a non-safety device.............. 1 2 3 4 5 N/A
5. The safety feature works well with a wide variety of hand sizes............................ 1 2 3 4 5 N/A
6. The safety feature works with a butterfly... 1 2 3 4 5 N/A
7. A clear and unmistakable change (either audible or visible) occurs when the
   safety feature is activated... 1 2 3 4 5 N/A
8. The safety feature operates reliably... 1 2 3 4 5 N/A
9. The exposed sharp is blunted or covered after use and prior to disposal................ 1 2 3 4 5 N/A
10. The inner vacuum tube needle (rubber sleeved needle) **does not** present a
    danger of exposure.. 1 2 3 4 5 N/A
11. The **product does** not need extensive training to be operated correctly.................1 2 3 4 5 N/A

Of the above questions, which three are the most important to **your** safety when using this product?

Are there other questions which you feel should be asked regarding the safety/ utility of this product?

Punctur-Guard Winged Set for Blood Collection

Device Description:
The Punctur-Guard Winged Set for Blood Collection or Infusion uses in-the-vein blunting technology to provide the highest level of needlestick prevention available.

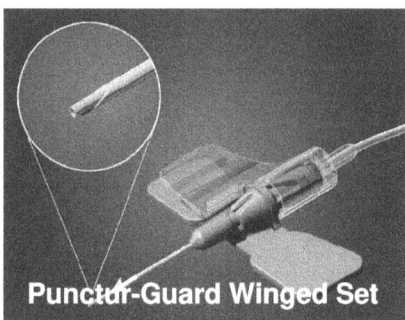

Punctur-Guard Winged Set

Advantages:
The Punctur-Guard in-the-vein blunting tehcnology allows the clinician to render the device safe prior to removing it from the patient's vein, therefore eliminating the risk of exposure to a contaminated sharps. It is the only Winged Set that is rendered safe immediately upon insertion in the vein and remains safe during the entire procedure until disposal. The Punctur-Guard Winged Set is also FDA approved for short term infusion.

Safety Features and Benefits:
In-the-vein blunting technology

FDA Status:	Approved
Sizes Available:	25G, 23G, 21G, 19G
Product Website:	http://www.icumed.com/Punctureguard.asp
Brochure Download:	http://www.icumed.com/Punctureguard.asp
Instructional Website:	http://www.icumed.com/Punctureguard.asp
Instructional Video:	http://www.icumed.com/Punctureguard.asp
Contact for Samples:	Visit the Medical Safety Book.com Sample Procurement Center
Contact for Purchase:	Contact ICU Medical, Inc.
Availability:	Now available
Manufacturer:	ICU Medical, Inc. 951 Calle Amanecer San Clemente, CA 92673 USA 949-366-2183 www.icumed.com aburcar@icumed.com

Blood Collection Equipment

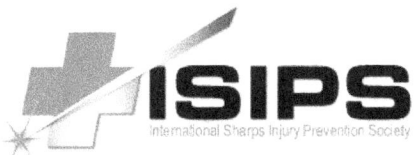

SAFETY WINGED NEEDLE EVALUATION FORM

Date: _____ Department: _____
Evaluator: _____ Product: _____ Number of times used: _____

Please **circle** the most appropriate answer for each question. Not applicable (N/A) may be used if the question does not apply to this particular product.

		Agree.........Disagree
1	The use of the Safety winged needle does not require extensive change in technique from the use of standard winged needles.	1 2 3 4 5 N/A
2	This device provides a better alternative to traditional winged needles.	1 2 3 4 5 N/A
3	This winged needle is no more difficult to use than traditional winged needles and requires no additional time.	1 2 3 4 5 N/A
4	The winged needle works well with a wide variety of hand sizes.	1 2 3 4 5 N/A
5	The winged needle is easy to handle while wearing gloves.	1 2 3 4 5 N/A
6	The winged needle can be used by either right or left handed clinicians.	1 2 3 4 5 N/A
7	The safety feature of the winged needle does not cause interference with the procedure.	1 2 3 4 5 N/A
8	The user does not need extensive training for correct use of the product.	1 2 3 4 5 N/A
9	The product is suitable for a range of uses across a variety of patient populations.	1 2 3 4 5 N/A
10	The safety feature of the product is a passive feature; it requires no intervention on the part of the clinician to activate.	1 2 3 4 5 N/A
11	The user's hands are protected from the sharp at all times.	1 2 3 4 5 N/A
12	The winged needle gives indication of safety feature activation.	1 2 3 4 5 N/A
13	The winged needle provides audible and visual feedback that the safety feature has been activated.	1 2 3 4 5 N/A
14	The winged needle has an undefeatable safety feature that provides permanent coverage of the sharp.	1 2 3 4 5 N/A
15	The winged needle operates reliably.	1 2 3 4 5 N/A
16	The design of the product suggests proper use.	1 2 3 4 5 N/A
17	The design of the safety winged needle allows it to be flush against skin without a high profile.	1 2 3 4 5 N/A
18	Use of the product requires you to use the safety feature.	1 2 3 4 5 N/A

Of the above questions, which three are the most important to your safety when using this product?

Are there other questions which you feel should be asked regarding the safety features of this product?

Conclusions: _____ -

Saf-T Holder® Devices

Device Description:
Saf-T Holder® devices are available with Saf-T Wing® Blood Collection Sets to facilitate blood collection with a vacuum tube. Saf-T Holder® devices also provide easy needleless transfer after a syringe draw.

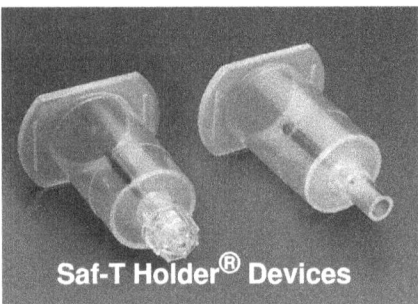

Saf-T Holder® Devices

Advantages:
Saf-T Holder® Devices come pre-attached to Saf-T Wing® Blood Collection sets. A special configuration of the Saf-T Holder® device for needleless blood transfer molds the syringe tip adapter fitting directly into the holder as one complete piece, providing easy compliance with OSHA directives for syringe draws.

Safety Features and Benefits:
Saf-T Holder® devices come with a pre-attached back-end needle and luer, eliminating exposures and holder re-use, compliant with OSHA directives. Saf-T Holder® devices also provide simple needleless blood transfers from a syringe after a controlled draw.

FDA Status:	Approved
Sizes Available:	Available for Saf-T Wing® Blood Collection Sets and needleless blood transfer.
Product Website:	www.smiths-medical.com
Brochure Download:	www.smiths-medical.com
Instructional Website:	www.smiths-medical.com
Instructional Video:	www.smiths-medical.com
Contact for Samples:	Visit the Medical Safety Book.com Sample Procurement Center
Contact for Purchase:	Phone:(800) 258-5361 Fax: (603) 352-3703
Availability:	Now available
Manufacturer:	Smiths Medical 10 Bowman Drive Keene, NH 03431 USA 800-258-5361 www.smiths-medical.com info@smiths-medical.com

smiths

Blood Collection Equipment

Safety Feature Evaluation Form
I.V. ACCESS DEVICES

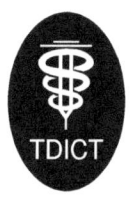

Date: _____ Department: _____ Occupation: _____

Product: _____ Number of times used: _____

Please **circle** the most appropriate answer for each question. Not applicable (N/A) may be used if the question does not apply to this particular product.

	agree............disagree
1. The safety feature can be activated using a one-handed technique.........................	1 2 3 4 5 N/A
2. The safety feature **does not** interfere with normal use of this product.....................	1 2 3 4 5 N/A
3. Use of this product requires you to use the safety feature.......................................	1 2 3 4 5 N/A
4. This product **does not** require more time to use than a non-safety device..............	1 2 3 4 5 N/A
5. The safety feature works well with a wide variety of hand sizes.............................	1 2 3 4 5 N/A
6. The device allows for rapid visualization of flashback in the catheter or chamber...	1 2 3 4 5 N/A
7. Use of this product **does not** increase the number of sticks to the patient...............	1 2 3 4 5 N/A
8. The product stops the flow of blood after the needle is removed from the catheter (or after the butterfly is inserted) and just prior to line connections or hep-lock capping..	1 2 3 4 5 N/A
9. A clear and unmistakable change (either audible or visible) occurs when the safety feature is activated..	1 2 3 4 5 N/A
10. The safety feature operates reliably...	1 2 3 4 5 N/A
11. The exposed sharp is blunted or covered after use and prior to disposal...............	1 2 3 4 5 N/A
12. The product **does not** need extensive training to be operated correctly..................	1 2 3 4 5 N/A

Of the above questions, which three are the most important to **your** safety when using this product?

Are there other questions which you feel should be asked regarding the safety/ utility of this product?

Saf-T Wing® Blood Collection Set

Device Description:
The Saf-T Wing® Blood Collection Set offers winged needle safety for delicate venous blood draws, utilizing a safety feature activated with a simple one- or two- handed technique. The Saf-T Wing® Blood Collection Set is available in three needle sizes, two tubing lengths, and with or without a pre-attached Saf-T Holder® device,

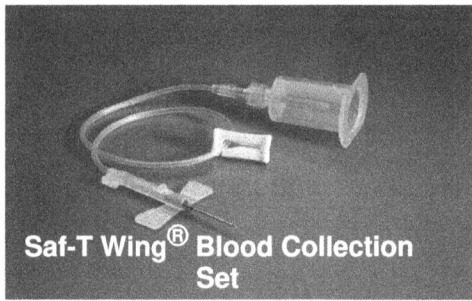

Saf-T Wing® Blood Collection Set

Advantages:
Saf-T Wing® Blood Collection Sets are available with a pre-attached Saf-T Holder® device. The Saf-T Wing® device can accommodate blood collection via either a vacuum tube or syringe. If there is a need to switch to a syringe at any time during the draw, the tubing can be clamped off, the holder removed, and a syringe secured to facilitate a controlled draw.

Safety Features and Benefits:
The Saf-T Holder® device which comes with the back-end needle and luer permanently attached to the holder, eliminates potential exposures and holder re-use, compliant with OSHA directives. The safety feature can be activated while the device is in the patient's arm, reducing needlestick exposure time.

Mechanics:
The safety feature can be activated with a one- or two-handed technique while still in the patient's arm.

FDA Status:	Approved
Sizes Available:	21, 23, 25g; 6" or 12" tubing
Product Website:	www.smiths-medical.com
Brochure Download:	www.smiths-medical.com
Instructional Website:	www.smiths-medical.com
Instructional Video:	www.smiths-medical.com
Contact for Samples:	Visit the Medical Safety Book.com Sample Procurement Center
Contact for Purchase:	Phone:(800) 258-5361 Fax: (603) 352-3703
Availability:	Now available
Manufacturer:	Smiths Medical 10 Bowman Drive Keene, NH 03431 USA 800-258-5361 www.smiths-medical.com info@smiths-medical.com

Blood Collection Equipment

smiths

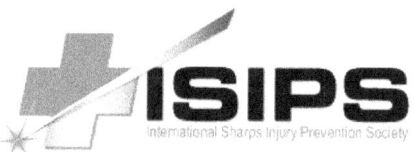

SAFETY WINGED NEEDLE EVALUATION FORM

Date: _____ Department: _____

Evaluator: _____ Product: _____ Number of times used: _____

Please **circle** the most appropriate answer for each question. Not applicable (N/A) may be used if the question does not apply to this particular product.

		Agree.........Disagree
1	The use of the Safety winged needle does not require extensive change in technique from the use of standard winged needles.	1 2 3 4 5 N/A
2	This device provides a better alternative to traditional winged needles.	1 2 3 4 5 N/A
3	This winged needle is no more difficult to use than traditional winged needles and requires no additional time.	1 2 3 4 5 N/A
4	The winged needle works well with a wide variety of hand sizes.	1 2 3 4 5 N/A
5	The winged needle is easy to handle while wearing gloves.	1 2 3 4 5 N/A
6	The winged needle can be used by either right or left handed clinicians.	1 2 3 4 5 N/A
7	The safety feature of the winged needle does not cause interference with the procedure.	1 2 3 4 5 N/A
8	The user does not need extensive training for correct use of the product.	1 2 3 4 5 N/A
9	The product is suitable for a range of uses across a variety of patient populations.	1 2 3 4 5 N/A
10	The safety feature of the product is a passive feature; it requires no intervention on the part of the clinician to activate.	1 2 3 4 5 N/A
11	The user's hands are protected from the sharp at all times.	1 2 3 4 5 N/A
12	The winged needle gives indication of safety feature activation.	1 2 3 4 5 N/A
13	The winged needle provides audible and visual feedback that the safety feature has been activated.	1 2 3 4 5 N/A
14	The winged needle has an undefeatable safety feature that provides permanent coverage of the sharp.	1 2 3 4 5 N/A
15	The winged needle operates reliably.	1 2 3 4 5 N/A
16	The design of the product suggests proper use.	1 2 3 4 5 N/A
17	The design of the safety winged needle allows it to be flush against skin without a high profile.	1 2 3 4 5 N/A
18	Use of the product requires you to use the safety feature.	1 2 3 4 5 N/A

Of the above questions, which three are the most important to your safety when using this product?

Are there other questions which you feel should be asked regarding the safety features of this product?

Conclusions: _____ -

SampLok® Sampling Kit

Device Description:
SampLok® Sampling Kit (SSK) is an OSHA-friendly platelet transfer kit. It provides accurate sample measurement as well as minimal platelet and biohazard waste.

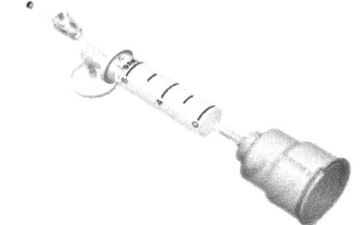

Advantages:
Advantages include the ability to streamline procedures with fewer steps to collect and transfer samples along with ease of use.

SampLok® Sampling Kit

Safety Features and Benefits:
Safety benefits include a reduced potential for needle stick injuries due to the included safety lid.

FDA Status:	Approved
Sizes Available:	N/A
Product Website:	www.itlcorporation.com
Brochure Download:	www.itlcorporation.com
Instructional Website:	www.itlcorporation.com
Instructional Video:	www.itlcorporation.com
Contact for Samples:	Visit the Medical Safety Book.com Sample Procurement Center
Contact for Purchase:	Purchase orders can be placed by fax at (703) 435-6700 or by email at sales@itlus.com
Availability:	Now available
Manufacturer:	ITL Corporation 1175 Herndon Parkway Suite 350 Herndon, VA 20170 USA 703-435-6700 www.itlcorporation.com sales@itlus.com

Blood Collection Equipment

SAFETY FEATURE EVALUATION FORM
I.V. ACCESS DEVICES

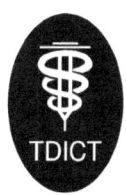

Date: _____ Department: _____ Occupation: _____

Product: _____ Number of times used: _____

Please **circle** the most appropriate answer for each question. Not applicable (N/A) may be used if the question does not apply to this particular product.

agree............disagree

1. The safety feature can be activated using a one-handed technique........................ 1 2 3 4 5 N/A
2. The safety feature **does not** interfere with normal use of this product..................... 1 2 3 4 5 N/A
3. Use of this product requires you to use the safety feature...................................... 1 2 3 4 5 N/A
4. This product **does not** require more time to use than a non-safety device.............. 1 2 3 4 5 N/A
5. The safety feature works well with a wide variety of hand sizes............................. 1 2 3 4 5 N/A
6. The device allows for rapid visualization of flashback in the catheter or chamber... 1 2 3 4 5 N/A
7. Use of this product **does not** increase the number of sticks to the patient...............1 2 3 4 5 N/A
8. The product stops the flow of blood after the needle is removed from the catheter (or after the butterfly is inserted) and just prior to line connections or hep-lock capping... 1 2 3 4 5 N/A
9. A clear and unmistakable change (either audible or visible) occurs when the safety feature is activated... 1 2 3 4 5 N/A
10. The safety feature operates reliably.. 1 2 3 4 5 N/A
11. The exposed sharp is blunted or covered after use and prior to disposal.............. 1 2 3 4 5 N/A
12. The product **does not** need extensive training to be operated correctly.................. 1 2 3 4 5 N/A

Of the above questions, which three are the most important to **your** safety when using this product?

Are there other questions which you feel should be asked regarding the safety/ utility of this product?

S-Monovette® Blood Collection System

Device Description:

The S-Monovette® is an enclosed multiple-sampling blood collection system that utilizes either an aspiration or vacuum method of collection. The aspiration method of collection virtually eliminates syringe draws and provides a closed connection for line draws. The system includes tubes in a full range of volumes and additives, multi-sampling needles with pre-assembled holders, needle protection devices, and safety winged blood collection sets.

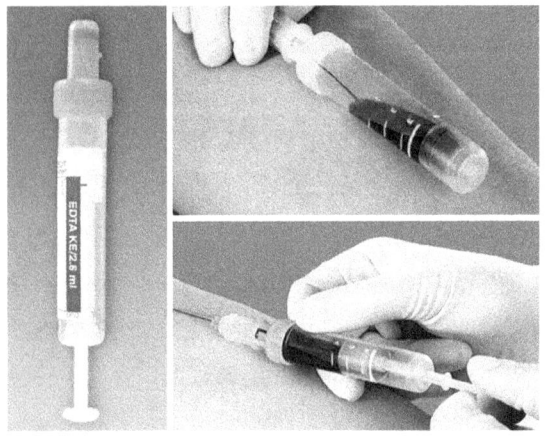

Advantages:

Aspiration method: The S-Monovette® and needle are assembled immediately prior to collection. After venipuncture, the plunger is withdrawn slowly until the tube is filled. Vacuum method: A vacuum is formed immediately prior to collection by locking the piston into the base of the S-Monovette® and breaking off the plunger. After the vein is punctured, the evacuated S-Monovette® is connected to the needle.

Safety Features and Benefits:

Using the S-Monovette® aspiration method of collection minimizes needlestick injuries by eliminating the practice of drawing blood from a vein or in-line system into a syringe and back sticking into a blood tube. The all-plastic screw cap tubes minimize breakage and the aerosol effect. The multi-sampling needles with pre-assembled holders are not reusable and prevent any risk of needlestick injury that may occur by unscrewing a contaminated needle from the holder.

FDA Status:	Other
Sizes Available:	Full range of volumes and additives
Product Website:	www.sarstedt.com/php/produktfamilie-darstellung.php?familie_id=111&seite=0
Brochure Download:	www.sarstedt.com/php/prospektanforderung.php?selected_gruppe_id=11
Instructional Website:	www.sarstedt.com/php/produktfamilie-darstellung.php?familie_id=111&seite=0
Instructional Video:	
Contact for Samples:	
Contact for Purchase:	(800) 257-5101; sarstedt@bellsouth.net; www.sarstedt.com/php/email.php
Availability:	Now available
Manufacturer:	Sarstedt, Inc. 1025 St. James Church Road P.O. Box 468 Newton, NC 28658 USA 800-257-5101 www.sarstedt.com sarstedt@bellsouth.net

Blood Collection Equipment

SARSTEDT

VACUUM TUBE BLOOD COLLECTION SYSTEMS

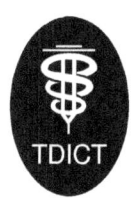

Date: _____ Department: _____ Occupation: _____

Product: _____ Number of times used: _____

Please **circle** the most appropriate answer for each question. Not applicable (N/A) may be used if the question does not apply to this particular product.

		agree............disagree
1.	The safety feature can be activated using a one-handed technique.........................	1 2 3 4 5 N/A
2.	The safety feature **does not** interfere with normal use of this product.....................	1 2 3 4 5 N/A
3.	Use of this product requires you to use the safety feature......................................	1 2 3 4 5 N/A
4.	This product **does not** require more time to use than a non-safety device..............	1 2 3 4 5 N/A
5.	The safety feature works well with a wide variety of hand sizes............................	1 2 3 4 5 N/A
6.	The safety feature works with a butterfly..	1 2 3 4 5 N/A
7.	A clear and unmistakable change (either audible or visible) occurs when the safety feature is activated...	1 2 3 4 5 N/A
8.	The safety feature operates reliably...	1 2 3 4 5 N/A
9.	The exposed sharp is blunted or covered after use and prior to disposal................	1 2 3 4 5 N/A
10.	The inner vacuum tube needle (rubber sleeved needle) **does not** present a danger of exposure...	1 2 3 4 5 N/A
11.	The **product does** not need extensive training to be operated correctly................	1 2 3 4 5 N/A

Of the above questions, which three are the most important to **your** safety when using this product?

Are there other questions which you feel should be asked regarding the safety/ utility of this product?

VACUETTE® QUICKSHIELD Safety Tube Holder

Device Description:
The QUICKSHIELD is a single-use plastic safety tube holder. Following venipuncture, a safety shield is activated to cover the needle and prevent accidental needlesticks.

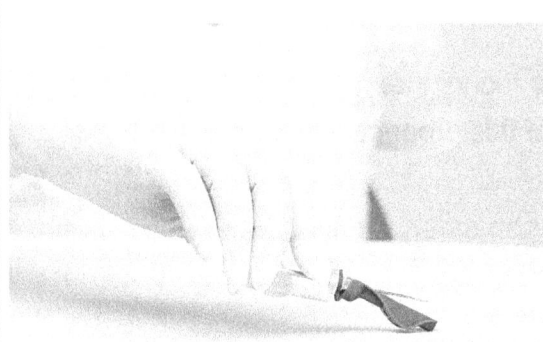

Simple, safe, practical

Advantages:
The QUICKSHIELD is remarkably easy to use. No change in blood collection technique is necessary. The holder is activated using only one hand to ensure immediate safety once the blood collection procedure is complete. Furthermore, the safety mechanism is activated in a smooth, easy to understand motion. An audible click indicates that the safety shield is in place.

Safety Features and Benefits:
Immediately following blood collection, the safety shield is activated by aid of a solid support. The fingers remain behind the needle tip throughout the procedure. The safety shield is attached firmly to the holder, and once the shield is activated, the needle is secure within the holder, and the holder is disposed of. Contact to blood is practically impossible.

FDA Status:	Approved
Sizes Available:	Short and long version
Product Website:	www.gbo.com
Brochure Download:	vacuette.gbo.com/en/support/3493.php
Instructional Website:	vacuette.gbo.com/en/support/3493.php
Instructional Video:	n/a
Contact for Samples:	Visit the Medical Safety Book.com Sample Procurement Center
Contact for Purchase:	As above
Availability:	Now available
Manufacturer:	Greiner Bio-One GmbH Bad Haller Str. 32 A-4550 Kremsmuenster, 4550 Austria 004-375-836-7910 www.gbo.com/preanalytics office@at.gbo.com

Blood Collection Equipment

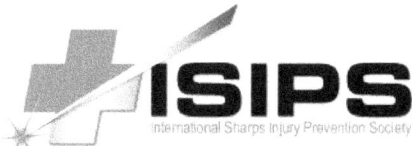

GENERIC SAFETY DEVICE EVALUATION FORM

Date: _____ Department: _____

Evaluator: _____ Product: _____ Number of times used: _____

Please **circle** the most appropriate answer for each question. Not applicable (N/A) may be used if the question does not apply to this particular product.

		Agree.........Disagree
1	The use of the device does not require extensive change in technique.	1 2 3 4 5 N/A
2	This device provides a better alternative to non-safety product.	1 2 3 4 5 N/A
3	This device is no more difficult to use than traditional non-safety product and requires no additional time.	1 2 3 4 5 N/A
4	The device works well with a wide variety of hand sizes.	1 2 3 4 5 N/A
5	The device is easy to handle while wearing gloves.	1 2 3 4 5 N/A
6	The device can be used by either right or left handed clinicians.	1 2 3 4 5 N/A
7	The safety feature of the device does not cause interference with the procedure.	1 2 3 4 5 N/A
8	The user does not need extensive training for correct use of the product.	1 2 3 4 5 N/A
9	The product is suitable for a range of uses across a variety of patient populations.	1 2 3 4 5 N/A
10	The safety feature of the product is a passive feature; it requires no intervention on the part of the clinician to activate.	1 2 3 4 5 N/A
11	The user's hands are protected from a sharp at all times.	1 2 3 4 5 N/A
12	The device gives indication of safety feature activation.	1 2 3 4 5 N/A
13	The device provides audible and visual feedback that the safety feature has been activated.	1 2 3 4 5 N/A
14	The device has an undefeatable safety feature that provides permanent coverage of the sharp.	1 2 3 4 5 N/A
15	The device operates reliably.	1 2 3 4 5 N/A
16	The design of the product suggests proper use.	1 2 3 4 5 N/A
17	Use of the product requires you to use the safety feature.	1 2 3 4 5 N/A
18	Use of the product removes a sharp thus removing potential for exposure to sharps injury and bloodborne pathogen exposure.	1 2 3 4 5 N/A

Of the above questions, which three are the most important to your safety when using this product?

Are there other questions which you feel should be asked regarding the safety features of this product?

Conclusions: _____

. _____

. _____

VACUETTE® Safety Blood Collection Set

Device Description:
The VACUETTE® Safety Blood Collection Set is a single-use, sterile, winged blood collection needle attached to flexible tubing (in various lengths). Also available with Luer Adapter or Luer Adapter and holder.

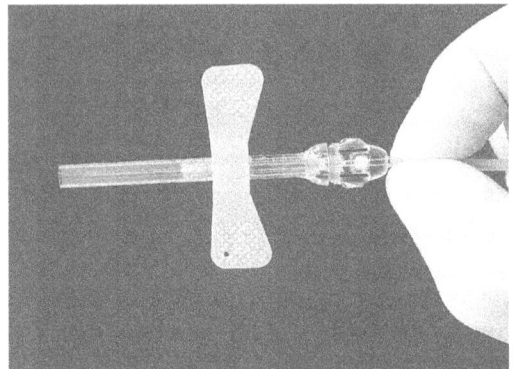

Many variations available

Advantages:
By using this product, safety is maximised for both blood collection personnel and patients. In particular, we can offer this product with the broadest range of variations; the ideal product for every application is available. The blood collection procedure is also made more comfortable, even for patients with difficult vein conditions. When blood collection is completed, the safety mechanism is easy to activate by pressing in both sides of the security lock.

Safety Features and Benefits:
Once the vein has been punctured correctly, blood flashback can be clearly seen through the translucent shield. After blood collection, the safety mechanism is activated within the vein, which means the risk window is minimal. Risk of needlestick injury is practically eliminated. The memory-free tubing is a further safety feature.

FDA Status:	Approved
Sizes Available:	21G, 23G, 25G
Product Website:	www.gbo.com
Brochure Download:	vacuette.gbo.com/en/support/3493.php
Instructional Website:	n/a
Instructional Video:	n/a
Contact for Samples:	
Contact for Purchase:	As above
Availability:	Now available
Manufacturer:	Greiner Bio-One GmbH Bad Haller Str. 32 A-4550 Kremsmuenster, 4550 Austria 004-375-836-7910 www.gbo.com/preanalytics office@at.gbo.com

Blood Collection Equipment

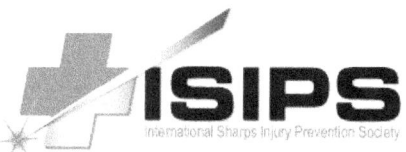

SAFETY WINGED NEEDLE EVALUATION FORM

Date: _____ Department:_____
Evaluator:_____ Product:_____ Number of times used:_____

Please **circle** the most appropriate answer for each question. Not applicable (N/A) may be used if the question does not apply to this particular product.

		Agree.........Disagree
1	The use of the Safety winged needle does not require extensive change in technique from the use of standard winged needles.	1 2 3 4 5 N/A
2	This device provides a better alternative to traditional winged needles.	1 2 3 4 5 N/A
3	This winged needle is no more difficult to use than traditional winged needles and requires no additional time.	1 2 3 4 5 N/A
4	The winged needle works well with a wide variety of hand sizes.	1 2 3 4 5 N/A
5	The winged needle is easy to handle while wearing gloves.	1 2 3 4 5 N/A
6	The winged needle can be used by either right or left handed clinicians.	1 2 3 4 5 N/A
7	The safety feature of the winged needle does not cause interference with the procedure.	1 2 3 4 5 N/A
8	The user does not need extensive training for correct use of the product.	1 2 3 4 5 N/A
9	The product is suitable for a range of uses across a variety of patient populations.	1 2 3 4 5 N/A
10	The safety feature of the product is a passive feature; it requires no intervention on the part of the clinician to activate.	1 2 3 4 5 N/A
11	The user's hands are protected from the sharp at all times.	1 2 3 4 5 N/A
12	The winged needle gives indication of safety feature activation.	1 2 3 4 5 N/A
13	The winged needle provides audible and visual feedback that the safety feature has been activated.	1 2 3 4 5 N/A
14	The winged needle has an undefeatable safety feature that provides permanent coverage of the sharp.	1 2 3 4 5 N/A
15	The winged needle operates reliably.	1 2 3 4 5 N/A
16	The design of the product suggests proper use.	1 2 3 4 5 N/A
17	The design of the safety winged needle allows it to be flush against skin without a high profile.	1 2 3 4 5 N/A
18	Use of the product requires you to use the safety feature.	1 2 3 4 5 N/A

Of the above questions, which three are the most important to your safety when using this product?

Are there other questions which you feel should be asked regarding the safety features of this product?

Conclusions: _____ -

VanishPoint® Blood Collection System

Device Description:
The VanishPoint blood collection system features a blood collection tube holder and a small diameter tube adapter. The needle is automatically retracted from the patient when the end-cap is closed after the last tube has been removed. This pre-removal activation virtually eliminates exposure to the contaminated sharp, effectively reducing the risk of needlestick injury. The tube adapter adapts a small collection tube to the VanishPoint blood collection tube holder.

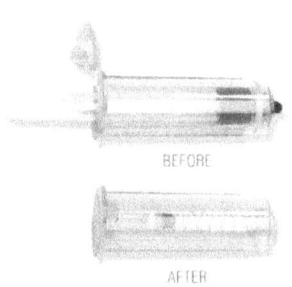

VanishPoint BCTH, Before & After

Advantages:
VanishPoint blood collection tube holders are compatible with standard, multiple sample blood collection needles. The user closes the end-cap of the VanishPoint blood collection tube holder after the last tube of blood has been removed. This automatically retracts the needle directly from the patient's vein into the barrel of the device, protecting the user from both ends of the contaminated sharp.

Safety Features and Benefits:
Since the needle is automatically retracted directly from the patient into the tube holder, exposure to the contaminated needle is virtually eliminated, effectively reducing the risk of needlestick injury. VanishPoint blood collection tube holders allow users to keep both hands behind the needle when activating the retraction mechanism. The single-use holder complies with safety regulations and prevents needle removal.

FDA Status:	Approved
Sizes Available:	Blood Collection Tube Holder, Small Diameter Tube Adapter
Product Website:	www.vanishpoint.com
Brochure Download:	www.vanishpoint.com/brochures.asp?section=purch
Instructional Website:	www.vanishpoint.com/instructionsBCTH.asp?section=hc and http://www.vanishpoint.com/instructionsSDTA.asp?section=hc
Instructional Video:	Available upon request
Contact for Samples:	Visit the Medical Safety Book.com Sample Procurement Center
Contact for Purchase:	(888) 703-1010, rtiservice@vanishpoint.com, or http://www.vanishpoint.com/rfi.asp?section=purch
Availability:	Now available
Manufacturer:	Retractable Technologies, Inc. 511 Lobo Lane Little Elm, TX 75068 USA 888-703-1010 www.vanishpoint.com rtisales@vanishpoint.com

Blood Collection Equipment

VANISHpoint

SAFETY FEATURE EVALUATION FORM
I.V. ACCESS DEVICES

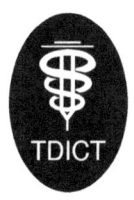

Date: _____ Department: _____ Occupation: _____

Product: _____ Number of times used: _____

Please **circle** the most appropriate answer for each question. Not applicable (N/A) may be used if the question does not apply to this particular product.

agree............disagree

1. The safety feature can be activated using a one-handed technique......................... 1 2 3 4 5 N/A
2. The safety feature **does not** interfere with normal use of this product.................... 1 2 3 4 5 N/A
3. Use of this product requires you to use the safety feature..................................... 1 2 3 4 5 N/A
4. This product **does not** require more time to use than a non-safety device.............. 1 2 3 4 5 N/A
5. The safety feature works well with a wide variety of hand sizes............................. 1 2 3 4 5 N/A
6. The device allows for rapid visualization of flashback in the catheter or chamber... 1 2 3 4 5 N/A
7. Use of this product **does not** increase the number of sticks to the patient...............1 2 3 4 5 N/A
8. The product stops the flow of blood after the needle is removed from the catheter (or after the butterfly is inserted) and just prior to line connections or hep-lock capping.. 1 2 3 4 5 N/A
9. A clear and unmistakable change (either audible or visible) occurs when the safety feature is activated.. 1 2 3 4 5 N/A
10. The safety feature operates reliably... 1 2 3 4 5 N/A
11. The exposed sharp is blunted or covered after use and prior to disposal.............. 1 2 3 4 5 N/A
12. The product **does not** need extensive training to be operated correctly................. 1 2 3 4 5 N/A

Of the above questions, which three are the most important to **your** safety when using this product?

Are there other questions which you feel should be asked regarding the safety/ utility of this product?

Venipuncture Needle-Pro® Device

Device Description:
The Venipuncture Needle-Pro® device is a holder-based safety device that is compliant with OSHA directives prohibiting needle removal. Portex® blood collection needles are available in a wide range of sizes and lengths and a variety of organizational bins and caddies are available for transport and storage.

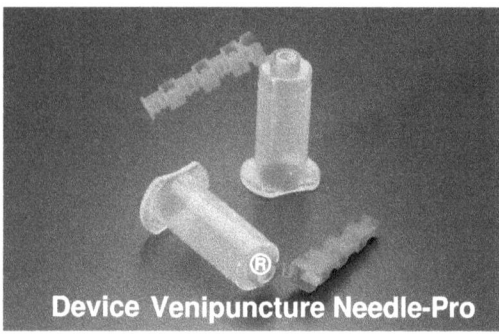

Device Venipuncture Needle-Pro

Advantages:
The holder-based design provides the clinician with added protection. The safety sheath can be rotated so the needle is in the desired "bevel up" position prior to venipuncture.

Safety Features and Benefits:
Because the Venipuncture Needle-Pro® device is a holder-based safety device, it prevents needle removal as per OSHA directives. This ensures that the holder will not be reused and eliminates potential back-end needle stick injuries.

Mechanics:
The orange hinged safety feature is activated with a simple one-handed technique against a hard surface.

FDA Status:	Approved
Sizes Available:	Available in bags of 1000, 10 bags of 100 and dispenser boxes of 25.
Product Website:	www.smiths-medical.com
Brochure Download:	www.smiths-medical.com
Instructional Website:	www.smiths-medical.com
Instructional Video:	www.smiths-medical.com
Contact for Samples:	
Contact for Purchase:	Phone:(800) 258-5361 Fax: (603) 352-3703
Availability:	Now available
Manufacturer:	Smiths Medical 10 Bowman Drive Keene, NH 03431 USA 800-258-5361 www.smiths-medical.com info@smiths-medical.com

smiths

Blood Collection Equipment

SAFETY FEATURE EVALUATION FORM
I.V. ACCESS DEVICES

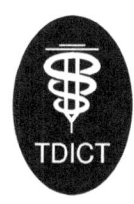

Date: _____ Department: _____ Occupation: _____

Product: _____ Number of times used: _____

Please **circle** the most appropriate answer for each question. Not applicable (N/A) may be used if the question does not apply to this particular product.

agree............disagree

1. The safety feature can be activated using a one-handed technique........................ 1 2 3 4 5 N/A
2. The safety feature **does not** interfere with normal use of this product.................... 1 2 3 4 5 N/A
3. Use of this product requires you to use the safety feature..................................... 1 2 3 4 5 N/A
4. This product **does not** require more time to use than a non-safety device.............. 1 2 3 4 5 N/A
5. The safety feature works well with a wide variety of hand sizes............................. 1 2 3 4 5 N/A
6. The device allows for rapid visualization of flashback in the catheter or chamber... 1 2 3 4 5 N/A
7. Use of this product **does not** increase the number of sticks to the patient...............1 2 3 4 5 N/A
8. The product stops the flow of blood after the needle is removed from the catheter (or after the butterfly is inserted) and just prior to line connections or hep-lock capping... 1 2 3 4 5 N/A
9. A clear and unmistakable change (either audible or visible) occurs when the safety feature is activated.. 1 2 3 4 5 N/A
10. The safety feature operates reliably... 1 2 3 4 5 N/A
11. The exposed sharp is blunted or covered after use and prior to disposal............... 1 2 3 4 5 N/A
12. The product **does not** need extensive training to be operated correctly................. 1 2 3 4 5 N/A

Of the above questions, which three are the most important to **your** safety when using this product?

Are there other questions which you feel should be asked regarding the safety/ utility of this product?

Blood Collection   Tubes-Plastic

Blood Sampling Systems

Blunt Tip Needle

Bone Marrow Collection

Bone Marrow Trays

The Compendium of
Infection Control Technologies

Medical Devices for Biomedical Safety

Blood Collection Tubes – Plastic -

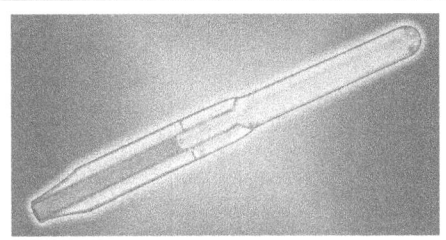

MicroSafe

MicroVette Capillary Blood Collection

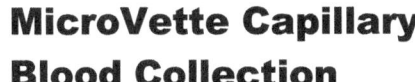

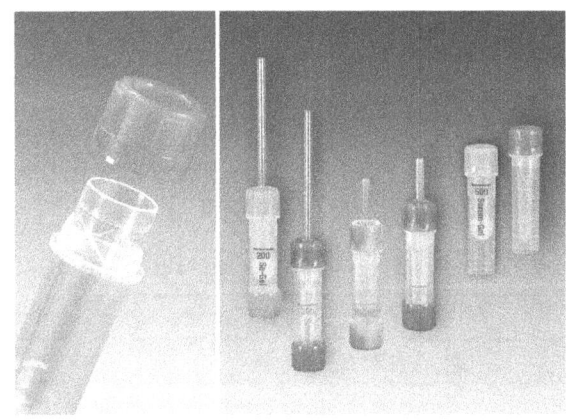

SampLok Tube Barrel Holder

S MonoVette Blood Collection System

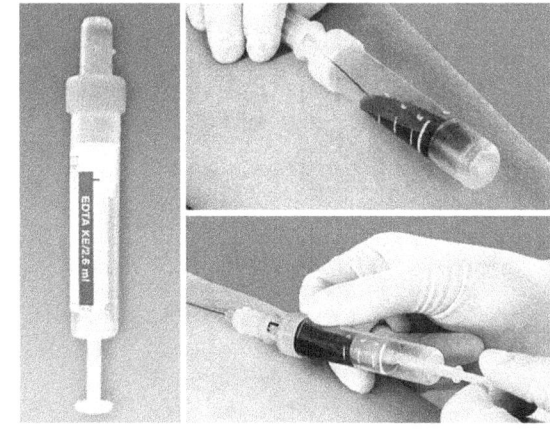

MICROSAFE®

Device Description:
One-piece, plastic tube used to collect and dispense whole blood from a finger-stick.

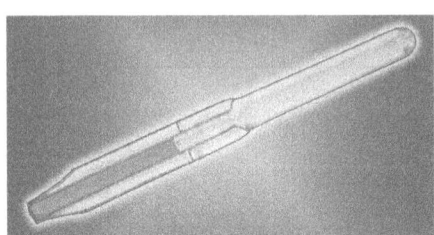

Advantages:
The MICROSAFE® tube fills automatically to a preset volume using capillary action. No aspiration… no air bubbles… no wasted samples. MICROSAFE® collection and dispensing tubes are available in volumes from 5 to 100 microliters.

Safety Features and Benefits:
Engineering controls designed to protect the healthcare worker - Plastic composition eliminates the need for hazardous glass collection devices - No chance of breakage
- No risk of injury.

Mechanics:
Easier to hold and manipulate - Ability to drop blood into solution with the use of one hand - Fills automatically via capillary action - Easier to dispense.

FDA Status:	N/A
Sizes Available:	5 to 100 microliters.
Product Website:	www.safe-tecinc.com
Brochure Download:	www.safe-tecinc.com/pdfs/microsafe.pdf
Instructional Website:	www.safe-tecinc.com/products.htm
Instructional Video:	
Contact for Samples:	
Contact for Purchase:	Please call 1-800-356-6033 for samples and ordering information.
Availability:	Now available
Manufacturer:	SAFE-TEC Clinical Products Inc. 142 Railroad Drive Ivyland, PA 18974 USA 215-364-5582 www.safe-tecinc.com aring@safe-tecinc.com

Blood Collection Tubes (Plastic)

JAFE-TEC
Clinical Products, Inc.

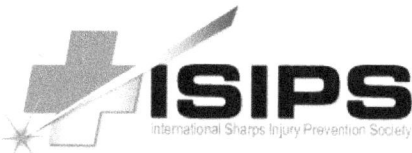

TUBES AND CONTAINERS EVALUATION FORM

Date: _____ Department:_____

Evaluator: _____ Product: _____ Number of times used: _____

Please **circle** the most appropriate answer for each question. Not applicable (N/A) may be used if the question does not apply to this particular product.

		Agree.........Disagree
1	The tube or container is made of plastic.	1 2 3 4 5 N/A
2	This device provides a better alternative to traditional product made out of glass.	1 2 3 4 5 N/A
3	This product is no more difficult to use than traditional winged needles and requires no additional time.	1 2 3 4 5 N/A
4	The product works well with a wide variety of hand sizes.	1 2 3 4 5 N/A
5	The product is easy to handle while wearing gloves.	1 2 3 4 5 N/A
6	The product can be used by either right or left handed clinicians.	1 2 3 4 5 N/A
7	The safety feature of the product does not cause interference with the procedure.	1 2 3 4 5 N/A
8	The user does not need extensive training for correct use of the product.	1 2 3 4 5 N/A
9	The product is suitable for a range of uses across a variety of patient populations.	1 2 3 4 5 N/A
10	The safety feature of the product is a passive feature; it requires no intervention on the part of the clinician to activate.	1 2 3 4 5 N/A
11	The user's hands are protected from a sharp at all times.	1 2 3 4 5 N/A
12	The product operates reliably.	1 2 3 4 5 N/A
13	The design of the product suggests proper use.	1 2 3 4 5 N/A
14	Use of the product requires you to use the safety feature.	1 2 3 4 5 N/A

Of the above questions, which three are the most important to your safety when using this product?

Are there other questions which you feel should be asked regarding the safety features of this product?

Conclusions: _____

_____

_____

Microvette® Capillary Blood Collection System

Device Description:
Sarstedt's Microvette® Capillary Blood Collection System is a safe and reliable system for the collection of 100 to 500µl. Microvette® 100 and 200, for 100 and 200µl volumes respectively, are designed with pre-assembled capillaries. Microvette® 300 and 500, for 300 and 500µl volumes respectively, are designed with special rims for the gravity flow principle of collection. Both versions have twist caps to minimize aerosols and are available in a full range of additives.

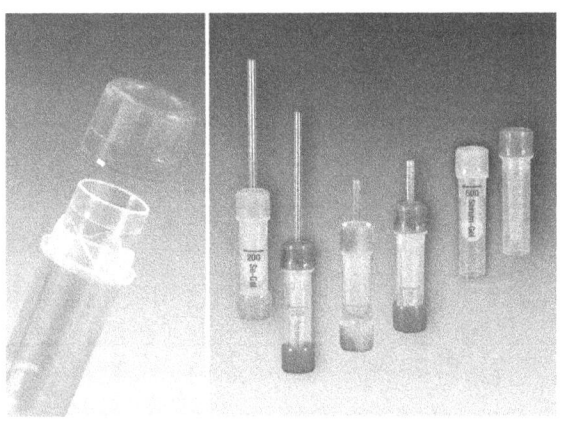

Advantages:
100 and 200µl: Collect blood until the assembled capillary is filled. Turn the tube upright to allow the blood to flow into the Microvette® tube. Turn the cap to remove and discard the pre-assembled capillary as one unit. Remove the cap from the base and seal the Microvette®. 300 and 500µl: Remove the twist cap and attach it to the base of the Microvette®. Collect blood using any part of the collection rim. Remove the cap from the base and seal the Microvette®.

Safety Features and Benefits:
Sarstedt's Microvette® Capillary Blood Collection System features an easy-to-use twist cap to reduce exposure to bloodborne pathogens via aerosols. Smooth tube interiors prevent sample hold-up, allowing optimal sample mixing and recovery.

FDA Status:	Listed
Sizes Available:	Full range of volumes and additives
Product Website:	www.sarstedt.com/php/produktfamilie-darstellung.php?familie_id=114&seite=0
Brochure Download:	www.sarstedt.com/php/prospektanforderung.php?selected_gruppe_id=11
Instructional Website:	www.sarstedt.com/php/produktfamilie-darstellung.php?familie_id=114&seite=0
Instructional Video:	
Contact for Samples:	
Contact for Purchase:	(800) 257-5101; sarstedt@bellsouth.net; www.sarstedt.com/php/email.php
Availability:	Now available
Manufacturer:	Sarstedt, Inc. 1025 St. James Church Road P.O. Box 468 Newton, NC 28658 USA 800-257-5101 www.sarstedt.com sarstedt@bellsouth.net

SARSTEDT

Blood Collection Tubes (Plastic)

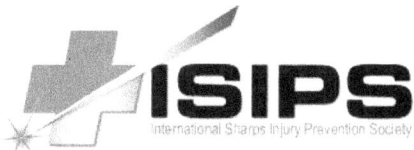

TUBES AND CONTAINERS EVALUATION FORM

Date: _____ Department: _____

Evaluator: _____ Product: _____ Number of times used: _____

Please **circle** the most appropriate answer for each question. Not applicable (N/A) may be used if the question does not apply to this particular product.

		Agree.........Disagree
1	The tube or container is made of plastic.	1 2 3 4 5 N/A
2	This device provides a better alternative to traditional product made out of glass.	1 2 3 4 5 N/A
3	This product is no more difficult to use than traditional winged needles and requires no additional time.	1 2 3 4 5 N/A
4	The product works well with a wide variety of hand sizes.	1 2 3 4 5 N/A
5	The product is easy to handle while wearing gloves.	1 2 3 4 5 N/A
6	The product can be used by either right or left handed clinicians.	1 2 3 4 5 N/A
7	The safety feature of the product does not cause interference with the procedure.	1 2 3 4 5 N/A
8	The user does not need extensive training for correct use of the product.	1 2 3 4 5 N/A
9	The product is suitable for a range of uses across a variety of patient populations.	1 2 3 4 5 N/A
10	The safety feature of the product is a passive feature; it requires no intervention on the part of the clinician to activate.	1 2 3 4 5 N/A
11	The user's hands are protected from a sharp at all times.	1 2 3 4 5 N/A
12	The product operates reliably.	1 2 3 4 5 N/A
13	The design of the product suggests proper use.	1 2 3 4 5 N/A
14	Use of the product requires you to use the safety feature.	1 2 3 4 5 N/A

Of the above questions, which three are the most important to your safety when using this product?

Are there other questions which you feel should be asked regarding the safety features of this product?

Conclusions: _____

_____

_____

_____

SampLok® Tube Barrel Holder

Device Description:
SampLok® Tube Barrel Holder facilitates safe inline blood sampling. SampLok® can be integrated with ITL's DonorCare® Needle Guard to provide additional protection from both the donor and sample needles.

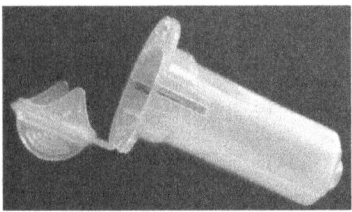

SampLok® with Hinged Lid

Advantages:
Advantages include compatibility for use with most current vacuum tubes, blood collection sets and luer adaptors, as well as a translucent material which allows visual sample collection.

Safety Features and Benefits:
The attached safety lid reduces risk of needle stick injury from sampling needles and improves safety for subsequent procedures.

FDA Status:	Approved
Sizes Available:	N/A
Product Website:	www.itlcorporation.com
Brochure Download:	www.itlcorporation.com
Instructional Website:	www.itlcorporation.com
Instructional Video:	www.itlcorporation.com
Contact for Samples:	Visit the Medical Safety Book.com Sample Procurement Center
Contact for Purchase:	Purchase orders can be placed by fax at (703) 435-6717 or by email at sales@itlus.com
Availability:	Now available
Manufacturer:	ITL Corporation 1175 Herndon Parkway Suite 350 Herndon, VA 20170 USA 703-435-6700 www.itlcorporation.com sales@itlus.com

Blood Collection Tubes (Plastic)

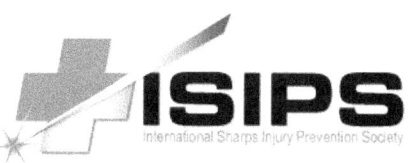

BLOOD DONOR PHLEBOTOMY DEVICE EVALUATION FORM

Date: _____ Department: _____

Evaluator: _____ Product: _____ Number of times used: _____

Please **circle** the most appropriate answer for each question. Not applicable (N/A) may be used if the question does not apply to this particular product.

		Agree.........Disagree
1	The safety feature does not obstruct vision of the tip of the needle.	1 2 3 4 5 N/A
2	This product does not require more time to use than a non-safety device.	1 2 3 4 5 N/A
3	Use of this product requires you to use the safety feature.	1 2 3 4 5 N/A
4	The safety feature works well with a wide variety of hand sizes.	1 2 3 4 5 N/A
5	The device is easy to handle while wearing gloves.	1 2 3 4 5 N/A
6	There is a clear and unmistakable change (audible or visible) that occurs when the safety feature is activated.	1 2 3 4 5 N/A
7	The safety feature operates reliably.	1 2 3 4 5 N/A
8	The needle is immediately shielded or retracted upon removal from vein.	1 2 3 4 5 N/A
9	The needle shielding is engaged from behind the needle.	1 2 3 4 5 N/A
10	After being placed in the permanently locked position the safety feature cannot be undone.	1 2 3 4 5 N/A
11	This safety product is no more difficult to use than non-safety products.	1 2 3 4 5 N/A
12	The user does not need extensive training for correct use of the product.	1 2 3 4 5 N/A
13	The design of the product suggests proper use.	1 2 3 4 5 N/A
14	It is not easy to skip a crucial step in proper use of the device.	1 2 3 4 5 N/A
15	The product can be easily used in either hand.	1 2 3 4 5 N/A
16	This device provides a better alternative to traditional blood donor phlebotomy devices.	1 2 3 4 5 N/A
17	The product is compatible for use with current blood collection sets produced by a variety of manufacturers.	1 2 3 4 5 N/A

Of the above questions, which three are the most important to your safety when using this product?

Are there other questions which you feel should be asked regarding the safety features of this product?

Conclusions: _____

_____

S-Monovette® Blood Collection System

Device Description:

The S-Monovette® is an enclosed multiple-sampling blood collection system that utilizes either an aspiration or vacuum method of collection. The aspiration method of collection virtually eliminates syringe draws and provides a closed connection for line draws. The system includes tubes in a full range of volumes and additives, multi-sampling needles with pre-assembled holders, needle protection devices, and safety winged blood collection sets.

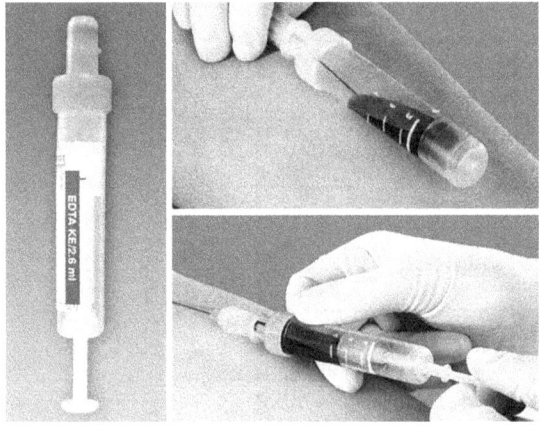

Advantages:

Aspiration method: The S-Monovette® and needle are assembled immediately prior to collection. After venipuncture, the plunger is withdrawn slowly until the tube is filled. Vacuum method: A vacuum is formed immediately prior to collection by locking the piston into the base of the S-Monovette® and breaking off the plunger. After the vein is punctured, the evacuated S-Monovette® is connected to the needle.

Safety Features and Benefits:

Using the S-Monovette® aspiration method of collection minimizes needlestick injuries by eliminating the practice of drawing blood from a vein or in-line system into a syringe and back sticking into a blood tube. The all-plastic screw cap tubes minimize breakage and the aerosol effect. The multi-sampling needles with pre-assembled holders are not reusable and prevent any risk of needlestick injury that may occur by unscrewing a contaminated needle from the holder.

FDA Status:	Other
Sizes Available:	Full range of volumes and additives
Product Website:	www.sarstedt.com/php/produktfamilie-darstellung.php?familie_id=111&seite=0
Brochure Download:	www.sarstedt.com/php/prospektanforderung.php?selected_gruppe_id=11
Instructional Website:	www.sarstedt.com/php/produktfamilie-darstellung.php?familie_id=111&seite=0
Instructional Video:	
Contact for Samples:	
Contact for Purchase:	(800) 257-5101; sarstedt@bellsouth.net; www.sarstedt.com/php/email.php
Availability:	Now available
Manufacturer:	Sarstedt, Inc. 1025 St. James Church Road P.O. Box 468 Newton, NC 28658 USA 800-257-5101 www.sarstedt.com sarstedt@bellsouth.net

SARSTEDT

Blood Collection Tubes (Plastic)

SAFETY FEATURE EVALUATION FORM
I.V. ACCESS DEVICES

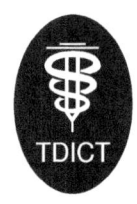

Date: _____ Department: _____ Occupation: _____

Product: _____ Number of times used: _____

Please **circle** the most appropriate answer for each question. Not applicable (N/A) may be used if the question does not apply to this particular product.

agree............disagree

1. The safety feature can be activated using a one-handed technique......................... 1 2 3 4 5 N/A
2. The safety feature **does not** interfere with normal use of this product..................... 1 2 3 4 5 N/A
3. Use of this product requires you to use the safety feature...................................... 1 2 3 4 5 N/A
4. This product **does not** require more time to use than a non-safety device.............. 1 2 3 4 5 N/A
5. The safety feature works well with a wide variety of hand sizes............................. 1 2 3 4 5 N/A
6. The device allows for rapid visualization of flashback in the catheter or chamber... 1 2 3 4 5 N/A
7. Use of this product **does not** increase the number of sticks to the patient...............1 2 3 4 5 N/A
8. The product stops the flow of blood after the needle is removed from the catheter (or after the butterfly is inserted) and just prior to line connections or hep-lock capping.. 1 2 3 4 5 N/A
9. A clear and unmistakable change (either audible or visible) occurs when the safety feature is activated... 1 2 3 4 5 N/A
10. The safety feature operates reliably... 1 2 3 4 5 N/A
11. The exposed sharp is blunted or covered after use and prior to disposal............... 1 2 3 4 5 N/A
12. The product **does not** need extensive training to be operated correctly.................. 1 2 3 4 5 N/A

Of the above questions, which three are the most important to **your** safety when using this product?

Are there other questions which you feel should be asked regarding the safety/ utility of this product?

Medical Devices for Biomedical Safety

Blood Sampling Systems

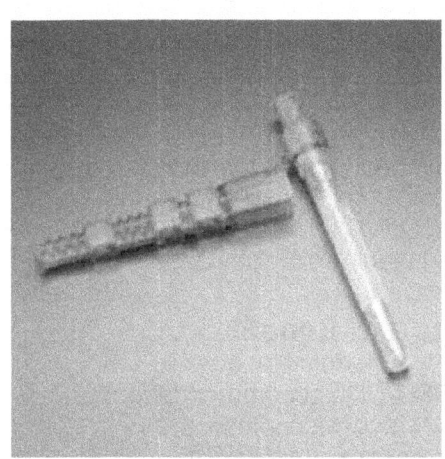

Blood Draw Hypodermic Peedle-Pro device

S MonoVette Blood Collection System

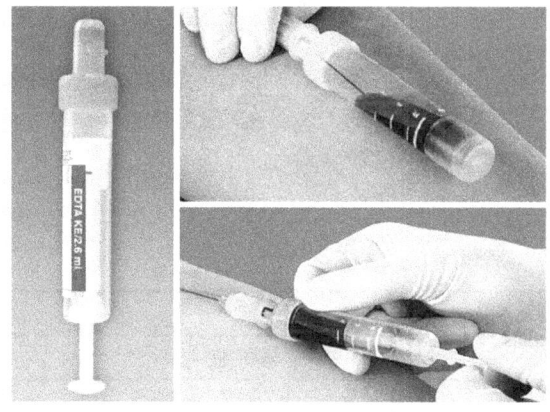

Blood Draw Hypodermic Needle-Pro® device

Device Description:
The Blood Draw Hypodermic Needle-Pro® device provides safety for controlled venous blood draws. Compatible with Luer slip and Luer lock syringes, the device is available with 20 – 25g needles ranging in length from ½" to 1 ½". Saf-T Holder® devices provide easy needleless transfer after the draw.

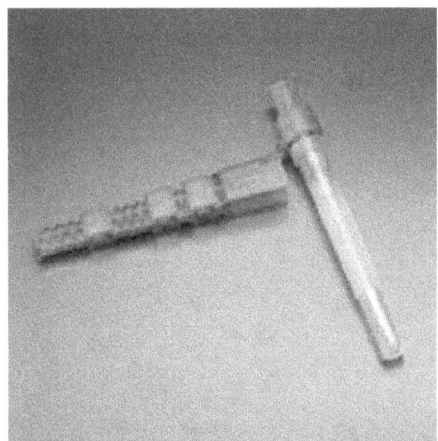

Blood Draw Hypodermic Needle-Pro®

Advantages:
Luer slip needle connections on the device allow for correct bevel positioning prior to the draw. Activation of safety feature is consistent with all Needle-Pro® devices.

Safety Features and Benefits:
The Blood Draw Hypodermic Needle-Pro® device meets NIOSH-CDC recommendations for safety devices. The device allows the user to control the venous draw with a syringe to prevent vein collapse. Activation of the safety feature is similar to all Hypodermic Needle-Pro® devices, reducing training.

Mechanics:
The Blood Draw Hypodermic Needle-Pro® Device is activated with a simple one-handed technique against any hard surface.

FDA Status:	Approved
Sizes Available:	20-25g; 1 ½" – 1"
Product Website:	www.smiths-medical.com
Brochure Download:	www.smiths-medical.com
Instructional Website:	www.smiths-medical.com
Instructional Video:	www.smiths-medical.com
Contact for Samples:	
Contact for Purchase:	Phone:(800) 258-5361 Fax: (603) 352-3703
Availability:	Now available
Manufacturer:	Smiths Medical 10 Bowman Drive Keene, NH 03431 USA 800-258-5361 www.smiths-medical.com info@smiths-medical.com

Blood Sampling Systems

smiths

SAFETY FEATURE EVALUATION FORM
SAFETY SYRINGES (and safety needles)

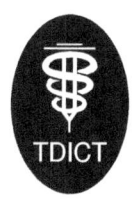

Date: —————— Department: —————————— Occupation: ——————————

Product: ———————————————————— Number of times used: ———————

Please **circle** the most appropriate answer for each question. Not applicable (N/A) may be used if the question does not apply to this particular product.

DURING USE: agree............disagree

1. The safety feature can be activated using a one-handed technique............1 2 3 4 5 N/A
2. The safety feature **does not** obstruct vision of the tip of the sharp............1 2 3 4 5 N/A
3. Use of this product requires you to use the safety feature.........................1 2 3 4 5 N/A
4. This product does not require more time to use than a non-safety device.................1 2 3 4 5 N/A
5. The safety feature works well with a wide variety of hand sizes................1 2 3 4 5 N/A
6. The device is easy to handle while wearing gloves...................................... 1 2 3 4 5 N/A
7. This device **does not** interfere with uses that do not require a needle......................1 2 3 4 5 N/A
8. This device offers a good view of any aspirated fluid..................................1 2 3 4 5 N/A
9. This device will work with all required syringe and needle sizes............... 1 2 3 4 5 N/A
10. This device provides a better alternative to traditional recapping.............. 1 2 3 4 5 N/A

AFTER USE:

11. There is a clear and unmistakeable change (audible or visible) that occurs
    when the safety feature is activated... 1 2 3 4 5 N/A
12. The safety feature operates reliably.. 1 2 3 4 5 N/A
13. The exposed sharp is permanently blunted or covered after use and prior to disposal.. 1 2 3 4 5 N/A
14. This device is no more difficult to process after use than non-safety devices........... 1 2 3 4 5 N/A

TRAINING:

15. The user **does not** need extensive training for correct operation............................. 1 2 3 4 5 N/A
16. The design of the device suggests proper use..1 2 3 4 5 N/A
17. It is **not** easy to skip a crucial step in proper use of the device.................................1 2 3 4 5 N/A

Of the above questions, which three are the most important to **your** safety when using this product?

Are there other questions which you feel should be asked regarding the safety/ utility of this product?

S-Monovette® Blood Collection System

Device Description:

The S-Monovette® is an enclosed multiple-sampling blood collection system that utilizes either an aspiration or vacuum method of collection. The aspiration method of collection virtually eliminates syringe draws and provides a closed connection for line draws. The system includes tubes in a full range of volumes and additives, multi-sampling needles with pre-assembled holders, needle protection devices, and safety winged blood collection sets.

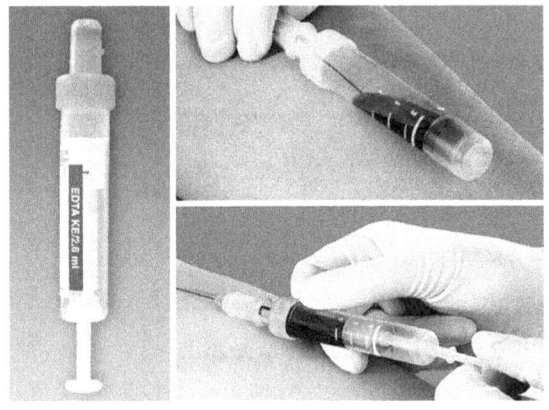

Advantages:

Aspiration method: The S-Monovette® and needle are assembled immediately prior to collection. After venipuncture, the plunger is withdrawn slowly until the tube is filled. Vacuum method: A vacuum is formed immediately prior to collection by locking the piston into the base of the S-Monovette® and breaking off the plunger. After the vein is punctured, the evacuated S-Monovette® is connected to the needle.

Safety Features and Benefits:

Using the S-Monovette® aspiration method of collection minimizes needlestick injuries by eliminating the practice of drawing blood from a vein or in-line system into a syringe and back sticking into a blood tube. The all-plastic screw cap tubes minimize breakage and the aerosol effect. The multi-sampling needles with pre-assembled holders are not reusable and prevent any risk of needlestick injury that may occur by unscrewing a contaminated needle from the holder.

FDA Status:	Other
Sizes Available:	Full range of volumes and additives
Product Website:	www.sarstedt.com/php/produktfamilie-darstellung.php?familie_id=111&seite=0
Brochure Download:	www.sarstedt.com/php/prospektanforderung.php?selected_gruppe_id=11
Instructional Website:	www.sarstedt.com/php/produktfamilie-darstellung.php?familie_id=111&seite=0
Instructional Video:	
Contact for Samples:	
Contact for Purchase:	(800) 257-5101; sarstedt@bellsouth.net; www.sarstedt.com/php/email.php
Availability:	Now available
Manufacturer:	Sarstedt, Inc. 1025 St. James Church Road P.O. Box 468 Newton, NC 28658 USA 800-257-5101 www.sarstedt.com sarstedt@bellsouth.net

SARSTEDT

Blood Sampling Systems

SAFETY FEATURE EVALUATION FORM
SAFETY SYRINGES (and safety needles)

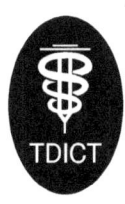

Date: ——————— Department: ——————————— Occupation: ———————————

Product: ———————————————————— Number of times used: ——————————

Please **circle** the most appropriate answer for each question. Not applicable (N/A) may be used if the question does not apply to this particular product.

DURING USE:
agree............disagree

1. The safety feature can be activated using a one-handed technique..........................1 2 3 4 5 N/A
2. The safety feature **does not** obstruct vision of the tip of the sharp............................1 2 3 4 5 N/A
3. Use of this product requires you to use the safety feature...1 2 3 4 5 N/A
4. This product does not require more time to use than a non-safety device.................1 2 3 4 5 N/A
5. The safety feature works well with a wide variety of hand sizes................................1 2 3 4 5 N/A
6. The device is easy to handle while wearing gloves..1 2 3 4 5 N/A
7. This device **does not** interfere with uses that do not require a needle....................1 2 3 4 5 N/A
8. This device offers a good view of any aspirated fluid...1 2 3 4 5 N/A
9. This device will work with all required syringe and needle sizes..............................1 2 3 4 5 N/A
10. This device provides a better alternative to traditional recapping............................1 2 3 4 5 N/A

AFTER USE:

11. There is a clear and unmistakeable change (audible or visible) that occurs
    when the safety feature is activated..1 2 3 4 5 N/A
12. The safety feature operates reliably...1 2 3 4 5 N/A
13. The exposed sharp is permanently blunted or covered after use and prior to dis-
    posal..1 2 3 4 5 N/A
14. This device is no more difficult to process after use than non-safety devices...........1 2 3 4 5 N/A

TRAINING:

15. The user **does not** need extensive training for correct operation............................1 2 3 4 5 N/A
16. The design of the device suggests proper use...1 2 3 4 5 N/A
17. It is **not** easy to skip a crucial step in proper use of the device...............................1 2 3 4 5 N/A

Of the above questions, which three are the most important to **your** safety when using this product?

Are there other questions which you feel should be asked regarding the safety/ utility of this product?

Medical Devices for Biomedical Safety
Blunt Tip Needles

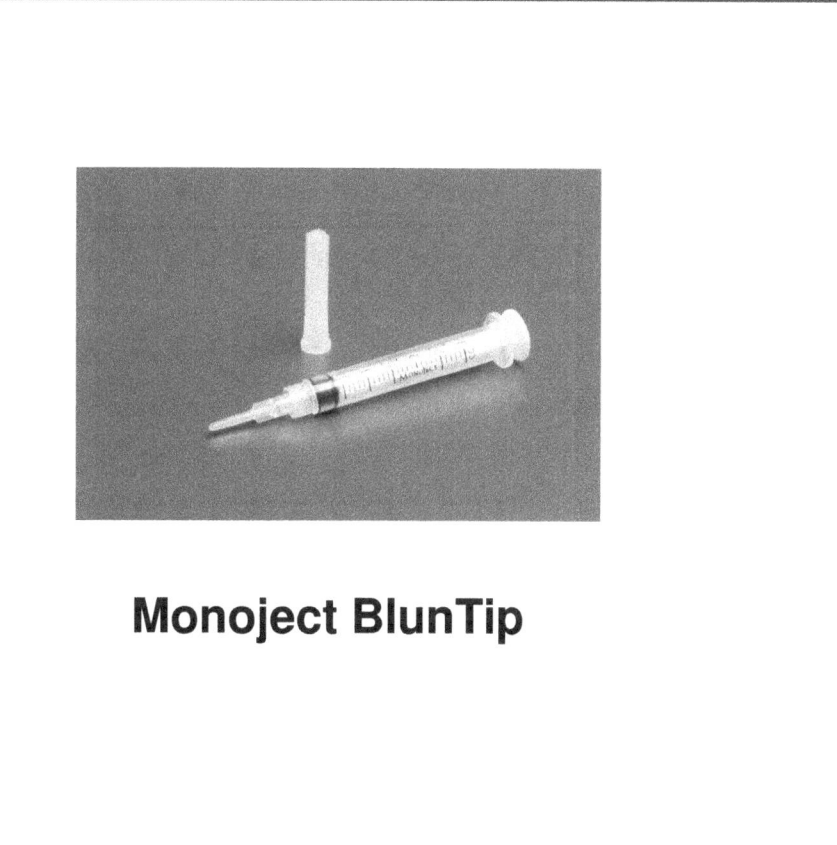

Monoject BlunTip

Monoject BlunTip

Device Description:
Plastic IV Access Cannual for use with Pre-Pierced Safety IV Ports. Also available with Vial Access device.

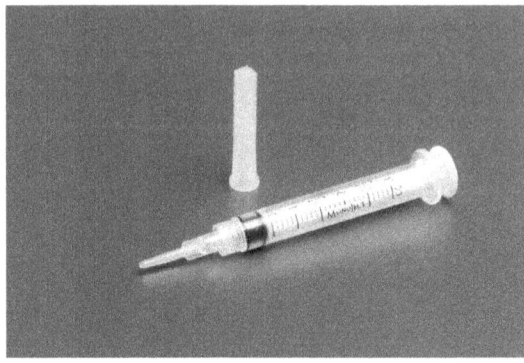

Advantages:
Latex Free, Blunt Plastic Cannula, Vial Access Cannula for easily accessing single-dose or multi-dose vials.

Safety Features and Benefits:
Complies with OSHA Bloodborne Pathogens Standard for Engineering Controls.Blunt Plastic Cannula virtually eliminates possible needlestick.

FDA Status:	Other
Sizes Available:	
Product Website:	www.tycohealthcare.com
Brochure Download:	www.tycohealthcare.com
Instructional Website:	www.tycohealthcare.com
Instructional Video:	www.tycohealthcare.com
Contact for Samples:	Visit the Medical Safety Book.com Sample Procurement Center
Contact for Purchase:	Contact your Kendall SharpSafety Representative.
Availability:	Now available
Manufacturer:	Tyco Healthcare/ Kendall
15 Hampshire Street
Mansfield, MA 02048
USA
508-261-6040
www.kendallhq.com
David.Clare@tycohealthcare.com

Blunt Needles

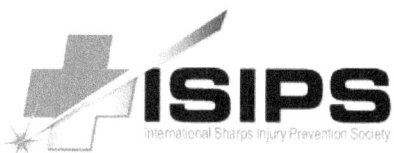

GENERIC SAFETY DEVICE EVALUATION FORM

Date: _____ Department: _____

Evaluator: _____ Product: _____ Number of times used: _____

Please **circle** the most appropriate answer for each question. Not applicable (N/A) may be used if the question does not apply to this particular product.

		Agree.........Disagree
1	The use of the device does not require extensive change in technique.	1 2 3 4 5 N/A
2	This device provides a better alternative to non-safety product.	1 2 3 4 5 N/A
3	This device is no more difficult to use than traditional non-safety product and requires no additional time.	1 2 3 4 5 N/A
4	The device works well with a wide variety of hand sizes.	1 2 3 4 5 N/A
5	The device is easy to handle while wearing gloves.	1 2 3 4 5 N/A
6	The device can be used by either right or left handed clinicians.	1 2 3 4 5 N/A
7	The safety feature of the device does not cause interference with the procedure.	1 2 3 4 5 N/A
8	The user does not need extensive training for correct use of the product.	1 2 3 4 5 N/A
9	The product is suitable for a range of uses across a variety of patient populations.	1 2 3 4 5 N/A
10	The safety feature of the product is a passive feature; it requires no intervention on the part of the clinician to activate.	1 2 3 4 5 N/A
11	The user's hands are protected from a sharp at all times.	1 2 3 4 5 N/A
12	The device gives indication of safety feature activation.	1 2 3 4 5 N/A
13	The device provides audible and visual feedback that the safety feature has been activated.	1 2 3 4 5 N/A
14	The device has an undefeatable safety feature that provides permanent coverage of the sharp.	1 2 3 4 5 N/A
15	The device operates reliably.	1 2 3 4 5 N/A
16	The design of the product suggests proper use.	1 2 3 4 5 N/A
17	Use of the product requires you to use the safety feature.	1 2 3 4 5 N/A
18	Use of the product removes a sharp thus removing potential for exposure to sharps injury and bloodborne pathogen exposure.	1 2 3 4 5 N/A

Of the above questions, which three are the most important to your safety when using this product?

Are there other questions which you feel should be asked regarding the safety features of this product?

Conclusions: _____

._____

._____

Medical Devices for Biomedical Safety

Bone Marrow Collection Systems

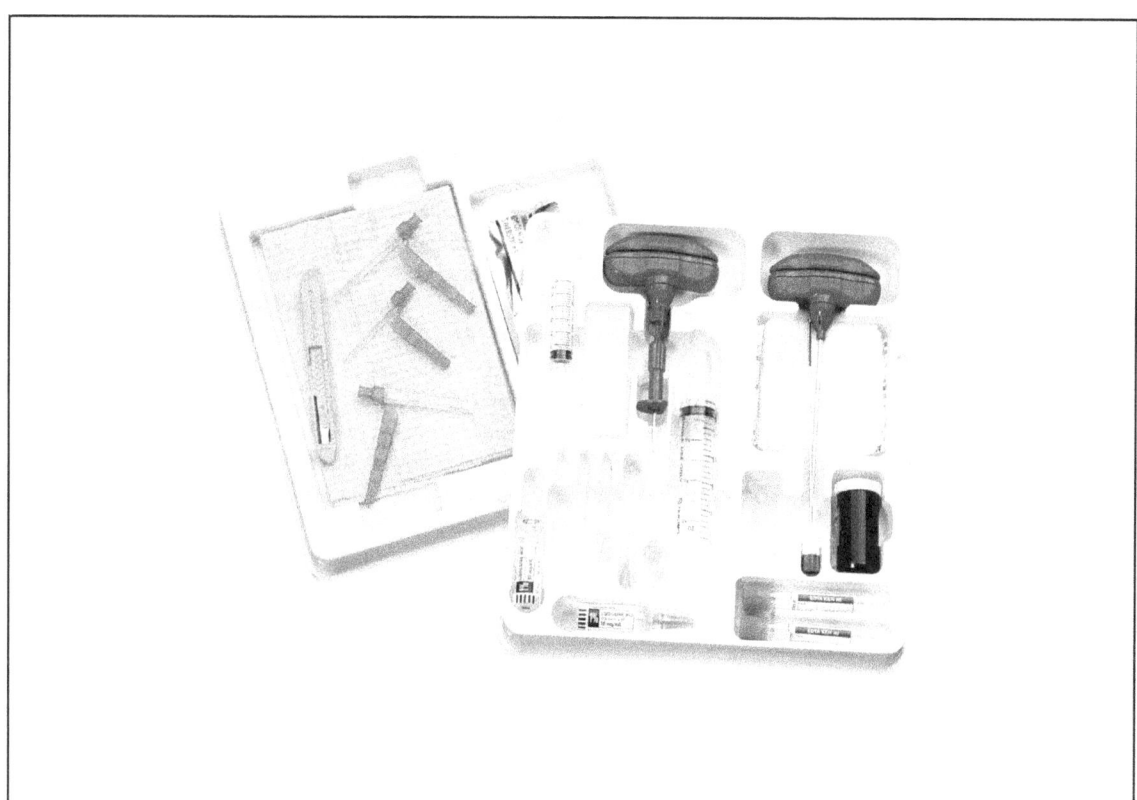

Jamshidi® Bone Marrow Biopsy/Aspiration Trays

Jamshidi® Bone Marrow Biopsy/Aspiration Trays

Device Description:

The Jamshidi® Bone Marrow Biopsy/Aspiration Needles and Marrow Acquisition Cradle (MAC) are designed to retrieve superior bone marrow biopsy samples with the protection of safety components. The MAC provides reliable specimen retention, offers greater patient comfort, eliminates painful redirects & allows for multiple sampling. The Cradle helps ensure user safety because it eliminates the need to remove the sample from the bone marrow needle through the sharp distal tip.

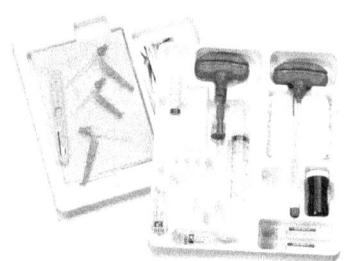

Advantages:

Versatile components for individual patient needs. The 2 pc. T-handle design provides increased control during needle insertion. A trocar-tapered stylet point and triple crown cannula tip provides a super sharp cutting edge for superior cortical penetration and medullary advancement that requires 25% less physical force. The MAC provides reliable specimen retention, greater patient comfort, eliminates painful redirects and allows for multiple sampling.

Safety Features and Benefits:

T-Handle Jamshidi® Bone Marrow Biopsy The Portex® Needle-Pro® Hypodermic System combines a hypodermic needle & protective sheath that covers the contaminated needle upon activation using a simple, one-handed technique. The Futura™ Safety Scalpel is used by depressing the inset to advance the exposed blade and depressing the inset again to activate blade retraction. The MAC (Marrow Acquisition Cradle) eliminates the need to remove the sample through the sharp distal tip.

Mechanics:

The Jamshidi is inserted into the marrow site using standard bone marrow biopsy procedure. Once a marrow core has been obtained in the device cannula, the Marrow Acquisition Cradle is used to safely capture the biopsy specimen by inserting the cradle into the proximal end of the biopsy needle prior to removal from the patient. The Marrow Acquisition Cradle allows removal of specimen from biopsy needle without sharp distal tip interaction.

FDA Status:	Approved
Sizes Available:	BCT3513 13G x 3.5"; BCT3411 11G x 4"; BAT3018 18G x 3"; BAT3015 15G x 3"; BCAT4511 11G x 4" & 15G x 3"; BCAT4508 8G x 4"; 15G x 3"; BCTM3411 11G x 4"; BCAM4511 11G x 4"; BCAM4508 8G x 4"; 15G x 3"
Product Website:	http://www.cardinal.com/mps/brands/specialprocedures/jamshidi.asp
Brochure Download:	N/A
Instructional Website:	N/A
Instructional Video:	N/A
Contact for Samples:	
Contact for Purchase:	To place an order, contact your Cardinal Health sales representative or call 800-964-5227.
Availability:	Now available
Manufacturer:	Cardinal Health 1430 Waukegan Rd. KB-B3 McGaw Park, IL 60085 USA 847-578-6457 www,cardinal.com linda.scott@cardinal.com

CardinalHealth

Bone Marrow Collection Systems

SAFETY FEATURE EVALUATION FORM
SAFETY SYRINGES (and safety needles)

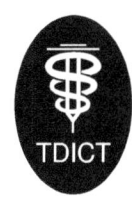

Date: —————— Department: —————— Occupation: ——————

Product: —————————————— Number of times used: ——————

Please **circle** the most appropriate answer for each question. Not applicable (N/A) may be used if the question does not apply to this particular product.

DURING USE:

agree............disagree

1. The safety feature can be activated using a one-handed technique............1 2 3 4 5 N/A
2. The safety feature **does not** obstruct vision of the tip of the sharp............1 2 3 4 5 N/A
3. Use of this product requires you to use the safety feature.......................1 2 3 4 5 N/A
4. This product does not require more time to use than a non-safety device.............. 1 2 3 4 5 N/A
5. The safety feature works well with a wide variety of hand sizes................. 1 2 3 4 5 N/A
6. The device is easy to handle while wearing gloves............................... 1 2 3 4 5 N/A
7. This device **does not** interfere with uses that do not require a needle............1 2 3 4 5 N/A
8. This device offers a good view of any aspirated fluid............................1 2 3 4 5 N/A
9. This device will work with all required syringe and needle sizes................ 1 2 3 4 5 N/A
10. This device provides a better alternative to traditional recapping.............. 1 2 3 4 5 N/A

AFTER USE:

11. There is a clear and unmistakeable change (audible or visible) that occurs
      when the safety feature is activated.. 1 2 3 4 5 N/A
12. The safety feature operates reliably.. 1 2 3 4 5 N/A
13. The exposed sharp is permanently blunted or covered after use and prior to disposal.. 1 2 3 4 5 N/A
14. This device is no more difficult to process after use than non-safety devices........... 1 2 3 4 5 N/A

TRAINING:

15. The user **does not** need extensive training for correct operation............................ 1 2 3 4 5 N/A
16. The design of the device suggests proper use... 1 2 3 4 5 N/A
17. It is **not** easy to skip a crucial step in proper use of the device................................ 1 2 3 4 5 N/A

Of the above questions, which three are the most important to **your** safety when using this product?

Are there other questions which you feel should be asked regarding the safety/ utility of this product?

Medical Devices for Biomedical Safety

Bone Marrow Trays

with Safety Components

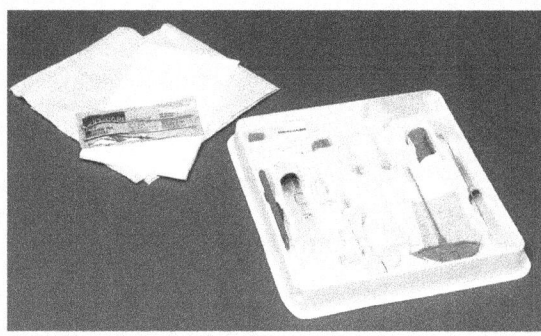

Monoject™ Bone Marrow Biopsy Trays

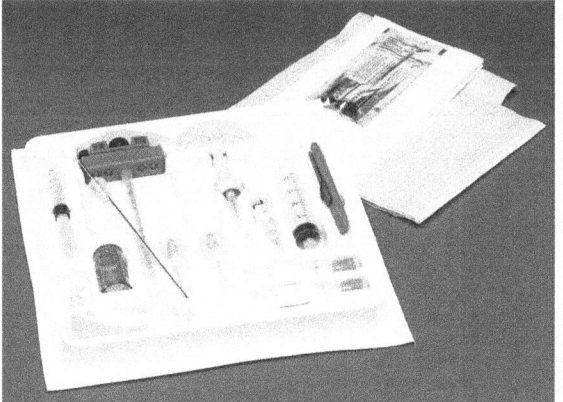

Snarecoil™ Bone Marrow Biopsy Trays

Monoject™ Bone Marrow Biopsy Trays

Device Description:
The Monoject™ Bone Marrow Biopsy/Aspiration Needle is ideal for obtaining a reliable aspirate and/or core bone marrow sample with unaltered architecture. The rigid stainless steel needle features a double-cutting edge cannula and sharp style for confident use and smoother entry into the marrow. The comfortable ergonomic handle design also provides precision control with minimal discomfort. Available as single needle and sterile tray configurations.

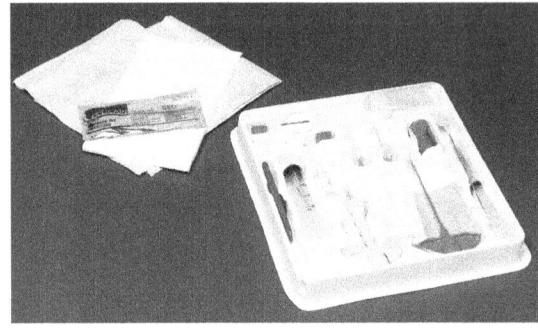

Advantages:
Each high quality procedure tray features Monoject™ Magellan safety needles, retractable scalpel blades and blunt tip aspiration needles.

Safety Features and Benefits:
Safety needles prevent accidental needlesticks.

Mechanics:
Each procedure tray comes with all components necessary to complete this procedure and features the Monoject Magellan Safety Needle.

FDA Status:	Approved
Sizes Available:	The single needles and trays come in a variety of sizes.
Product Website:	www.kendallhq.com
Brochure Download:	
Instructional Website:	
Instructional Video:	
Contact for Samples:	Visit the Medical Safety Book.com Sample Procurement Center
Contact for Purchase:	Contact your Local Sales Rep @ -800-962-9888. Product can also be ordered via your dealer of choice.
Availability:	Now available
Manufacturer:	Kendall Healthcare Marketing 15 Hampshire Street Mansfield, MA 02762 USA 508-261-8637 paula.girvan@tycohealthcare.com

Bone Marrow Trays with Safety Components

SAFETY FEATURE EVALUATION FORM
SAFETY SYRINGES (and safety needles)

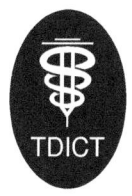

Date: —————— Department: —————————— Occupation: ——————————

Product: ————————————————— Number of times used: ——————————

Please **circle** the most appropriate answer for each question. Not applicable (N/A) may be used if the question does not apply to this particular product.

DURING USE:

agree............disagree

1. The safety feature can be activated using a one-handed technique...........................1 2 3 4 5 N/A
2. The safety feature **does not** obstruct vision of the tip of the sharp............................1 2 3 4 5 N/A
3. Use of this product requires you to use the safety feature...1 2 3 4 5 N/A
4. This product does not require more time to use than a non-safety device.................1 2 3 4 5 N/A
5. The safety feature works well with a wide variety of hand sizes................................1 2 3 4 5 N/A
6. The device is easy to handle while wearing gloves..1 2 3 4 5 N/A
7. This device **does not** interfere with uses that do not require a needle.......................1 2 3 4 5 N/A
8. This device offers a good view of any aspirated fluid...1 2 3 4 5 N/A
9. This device will work with all required syringe and needle sizes...............................1 2 3 4 5 N/A
10. This device provides a better alternative to traditional recapping............................1 2 3 4 5 N/A

AFTER USE:

11. There is a clear and unmistakeable change (audible or visible) that occurs
    when the safety feature is activated..1 2 3 4 5 N/A
12. The safety feature operates reliably...1 2 3 4 5 N/A
13. The exposed sharp is permanently blunted or covered after use and prior to disposal..1 2 3 4 5 N/A
14. This device is no more difficult to process after use than non-safety devices...........1 2 3 4 5 N/A

TRAINING:

15. The user **does not** need extensive training for correct operation.............................1 2 3 4 5 N/A
16. The design of the device suggests proper use...1 2 3 4 5 N/A
17. It is **not** easy to skip a crucial step in proper use of the device................................1 2 3 4 5 N/A

Of the above questions, which three are the most important to **your** safety when using this product?

Are there other questions which you feel should be asked regarding the safety/ utility of this product?

Snarecoil™ Bone Marrow Biopsy Trays

Device Description:
The Goldenberg Snarecoil line of Bone Marrow Biopsy Needles and Trays incorporates a unique and patented coil mechanism, eliminating the need to rock or sever the specimen. This revolutionary design helps clinicians to quickly harvest long, non-fragmented marrow needles. Available in single needles in a variety of sizes. Also packaged in sterile tray configurations to meet individual needs.

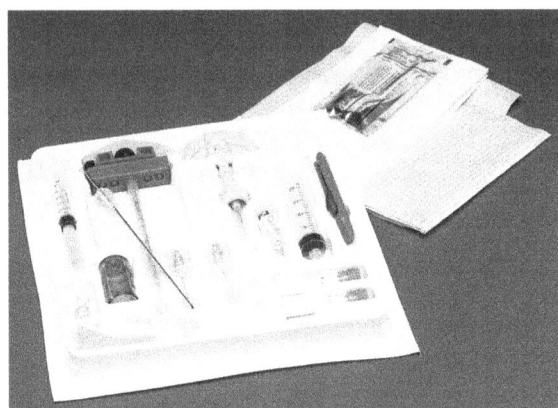

Advantages:
Each high quality procedure tray featues Monoject Magellan™ safety needles, retractable scalpel blades and blunt tip aspiration needles.

Safety Features and Benefits:
Safety needles prevent accidental needlesticks.

Mechanics:
Each procedure tray comes with all components necessary to complete the procedure and features the Monoject Magellan Safety Needle.

FDA Status:	Approved
Sizes Available:	Availabe in Single Needles and Trays.
Product Website:	www.kendallhq.com
Brochure Download:	
Instructional Website:	
Instructional Video:	
Contact for Samples:	Visit the Medical Safety Book.com Sample Procurement Center
Contact for Purchase:	Contact your Local Sales Rep @1-800-962-9888. Product can also be ordered via your dealer of choice.
Availability:	Now available
Manufacturer:	Kendall Healthcare Marketing 15 Hampshire Street Mansfield, MA 02762 USA 508-261-8637 paula.girvan@tycohealthcare.com

Bone Marrow Trays with Safety Components

SAFETY FEATURE EVALUATION FORM
SAFETY SYRINGES (and safety needles)

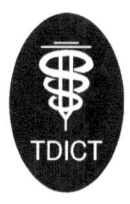

Date: —————— Department: ———————— Occupation: ——————————

Product: ————————————————— Number of times used: ——————————

Please **circle** the most appropriate answer for each question. Not applicable (N/A) may be used if the question does not apply to this particular product.

DURING USE:
agree...........disagree

1. The safety feature can be activated using a one-handed technique...........1 2 3 4 5 N/A
2. The safety feature **does not** obstruct vision of the tip of the sharp............1 2 3 4 5 N/A
3. Use of this product requires you to use the safety feature.........................1 2 3 4 5 N/A
4. This product does not require more time to use than a non-safety device................ 1 2 3 4 5 N/A
5. The safety feature works well with a wide variety of hand sizes...................... 1 2 3 4 5 N/A
6. The device is easy to handle while wearing gloves.............................. 1 2 3 4 5 N/A
7. This device **does not** interfere with uses that do not require a needle......................1 2 3 4 5 N/A
8. This device offers a good view of any aspirated fluid.............................1 2 3 4 5 N/A
9. This device will work with all required syringe and needle sizes............................... 1 2 3 4 5 N/A
10. This device provides a better alternative to traditional recapping.............................. 1 2 3 4 5 N/A

AFTER USE:
11. There is a clear and unmistakeable change (audible or visible) that occurs
     when the safety feature is activated... 1 2 3 4 5 N/A
12. The safety feature operates reliably... 1 2 3 4 5 N/A
13. The exposed sharp is permanently blunted or covered after use and prior to disposal.. 1 2 3 4 5 N/A
14. This device is no more difficult to process after use than non-safety devices........... 1 2 3 4 5 N/A

TRAINING:
15. The user **does not** need extensive training for correct operation............................ 1 2 3 4 5 N/A
16. The design of the device suggests proper use.. 1 2 3 4 5 N/A
17. It is **not** easy to skip a crucial step in proper use of the device................................ 1 2 3 4 5 N/A

Of the above questions, which three are the most important to **your** safety when using this product?

Are there other questions which you feel should be asked regarding the safety/ utility of this product?

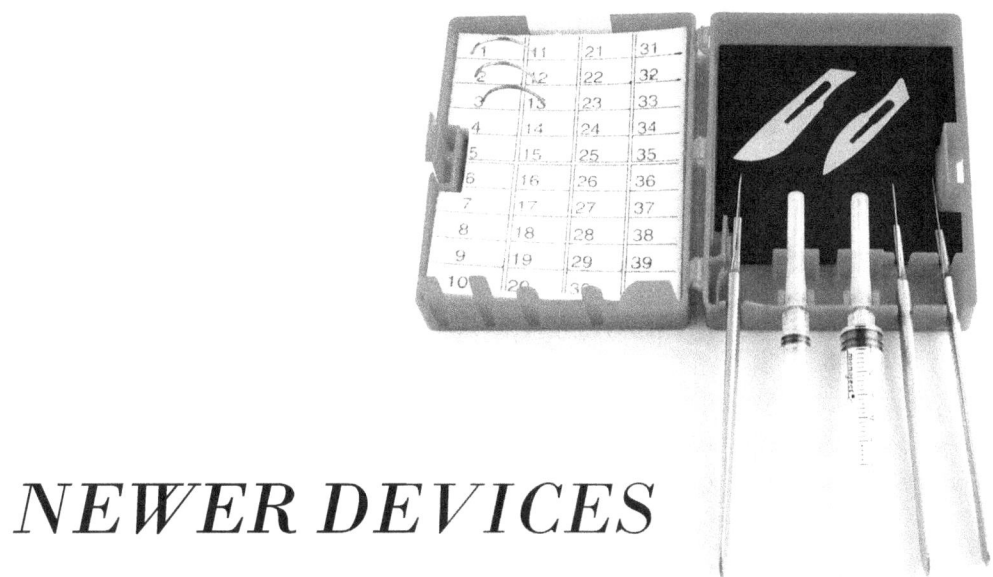

NEWER DEVICES

The devices on the following pages have been identified as currently available, but have not, as of this printing, been uploaded by their manufacturers.

The manufacturers have been contacted and most of them will be featured in the coming updates.

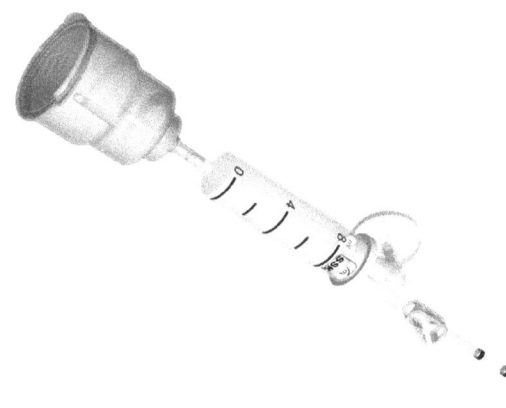

The following devices are the newer devices that fit into the above categories and the new categories that match alphabetically. We are currently waiting for their manufacturers to upload their descriptions and create their Compendium pages and choose their appropriate evaluation forms.

Make sure you join www.MedicalSafetyBook.com and we will notify you as soon as enough new devices have been

Air Bubble Removal Devices

Clinicians must expel air bubbles from blood samples safely without exposure to blood or bloodborne pathogens. Allows air out the filter end but does not allow blood. This device eliminates accidentally expelled blood droplets caused by aerosolizing air bubbles from a blood-filled syringe.

- Filter-Pro™ air bubble removal device; Smith's Medical, www.smiths-medical.com

Allergy Syringes

Allergen immunotherapy (allergy injection treatment) consists of repeated injections of one or more mixtures of extracts of allergens over a period of several years. A variety of allergy syringes are available with retractable needles, or shielded needles.

- SurGuard Safety Allergy Syringes and Trays; Terumo, www.terumotmp.com
- BD SafetyGlide™ Syringe for Allergy; BD, www.bd.com
- Hypodermic Needle-Pro® Safety Allergy Tray and needles; Smiths Medical, www.smiths-medical.com
- InviroSNAP! Safety Syringe Allergy Tray; Inviro Medical, www.inviromedical.com .
- MONOJECT™ Allergy Trays; Covidien, www.kendallsharpsafety.com
- VanishPoint® Allergy Syringe Tray and syringes; Retractable Technologies Inc., www.vanishpoint.com

Amniocentesis Trays

Amniocentesis is a procedure where fluid is aspirated out of the amniotic sac. Fetal urine, fetal cells, and various proteins move freely within this sac. During amniocentesis, a long needle is placed through the abdominal wall and into the amniotic sac. Once the needle is in the amniotic sac, a syringe is used to aspirate the amniotic fluid. The fluid is then sent for evaluation. New technologies provide safety sharps that can protect the user from needlesticks.

- Amniocentesis Tray; Smiths Medical, www.smiths-medical.com

Ampoule Breaker

Ampoules are small glass vessels in which liquids for injections are hermetically sealed. When the cap is snapped off, glass chips can fly off and a jagged or sharp edge can cut the hands of clinicians and others. The scoring at the neck does not always break where it is intended. This is due to the glass re-melding to some degree at the score line. In one study more than 62 percent of nurses said that they have been cut by a broken glass ampoule. Safety ampoule breakers prevent this problem by covering the glass ampoule during the breaking process, thus protecting the clinician's hands.

- Ampoule Breaker; Millipore Inc. www.millipore.com
- Ampoule Opener; Health Care Logistics, www.healthcarelogistics.com
- SafeBreaK™; Medi-Dose Inc., www.medidose.com
- Snapit™ Ampoule Opener; Qlicksmart, www.qlicksmart.com
- DAB Disposable Ampoule Breakers, Star Systems LLC, www.starrsystemsllc.com/
- Ampoule Adapters; West Pharmaceutical; www.westreconstitution.com

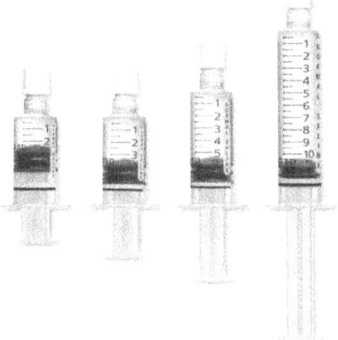

Anesthesia Trays

anesthesia trays containing safety-engineered components that minimize sharps injury potential.

- BD™ Anesthesia Safety Trays; BD; www.bd.com

Apheresis Needles

Apheresis is a special blood donation procedure in which plasma or selected cellular elements, such as platelets or white cells, are separated from the other parts of the blood and retained. Blood is drawn and processed through a cell separator, and the other cells and plasma are returned to the body. Apheresis takes approximately two hours compared with a whole blood donation of about eight to 10 minutes. During apheresis, the patient or donor is connected to the apheresis machine. A needle is inserted into a vein in each arm. Blood is withdrawn from one arm, run through the machine to extract the stem cells, and all the remaining components of the blood are returned to the donor through the needle in the other arm. In the case of a patient donating their own stem cells, this process is performed using a central venous catheter, which has two lumens.

- ITL Playtypus® Needle Guard - for use with Apheresis and AV Fistula needles, [available outside of the United States], ITL, www.itlcorporation.com/platypus.php
- MasterGuard Anti-Stick Needle Protector; Medic Anti-Stick Needle/Connector; Medisystems Corp; www.medisystems.com

- Nipro SafeTouch II Fistula Needles; Rockwell Medical Technologies Inc.,www.rockwellmed.com
- SysLoc Safety A.V. Fistula Needle Set, WingEaster A.V. Fistula Needle Guard; JMS North America Corporation, www.jmsna.net

Arterial Blood Gas Syringes

Arterial blood must be used for ABG measurement rather than venous blood because only arterial blood accurately reflects the amount of pO2 transferred from the lungs. Specialized safety products are used for this.

- Micro ABG Arterial Blood Gas Sampling Kits, Quik ABG Syringes; Vital Signs, Inc., www2.vitalsigns.com/VSIHome/html/english/default.aspx
- Pulset ABG Syringe; Westmed Inc., www.westmedinc.com
- safePICO Self-Filling Arterial Sampler, Radiometer America Inc., www.radiometeramerica.com

Arterial Catheter Stabilization Products

Arterial catheter stabilization products are designed to hold arterial lines in place throughout therapy. Rather than using sutures, with the inherent suture wounds and the potential for accidental needlesticks—just stabilization.

- Statlock Arterial Stabilization Device; CR Bard, www.statlock.com
- Zefon Arterial Anchor Bandage; Zefon International Inc., www.zefon.com

Arterial Line Draw

Arterial and venous infusion lines are used to introduce fluids into the blood stream of a patient. Typically the injection site is also used to take periodic blood samples from the patient.

- Deltran® Plus closed needleless arterial blood collection system; Utah Medical Products, www.utahmed.com/deltranplus.htm
- Venous Arterial blood Management Protection (VAMP) Plus, Vamp Adult, Vamp Jr.; Edwards Life Sciences, www.edwards.com
- Portex® Line Draw Plus and Umbilical Line Draw; Smiths Medical, www.smiths-medical.com.

Automated Filling of IV Syringe Doses

The standard method of filling syringes manually creates many opportunities of accidental needlesticks and other occupational exposure to medications. Automated systems are available that make the filling of syringes safer.

- Exacta-Mix™ 2400 Compounder (EM2400), Rapid-Fill™ Automated Syringe Filler (ASF); Baxa, www.baxa.com

Bifurcated Needles

Bifurcated needles administer vaccines by the scarification method. There is currently only one safety bifurcated needle available for smallpox vaccinations if they become necessary again.

- BD Eclipse™ Bifurcated Needle; BD, www.bd.com

Biohazard Spill Kit

A BioHazard Spill Clean-Up Kit provides everything necessary for cleanup of bodily fluids such as blood, vomit, urine etc.

- Sharps Biohazard Spill Cleanup and Disposal Kit - Disposal By Mail System; Sharps Compliance, Inc,; www.sharpsinc.com

Bleeding Time Devices

Bleeding time products make an incision and are then discarded into an approved sharps container. A timer is started and the edge of the incision is blotted at 30-second intervals with filter paper. The time that the bleeding stops is noted.

- Surgicutt® bleeding time; International Technidyne Corporation (ITC), a subsidiary of Thoratec Corporation, www.itcmed.com

Blood Collection

Blood drawing is the process of obtaining a sample of venous blood to assist in diagnosis. Typically a 5 ml to 25 ml sample of blood is adequate depending on what blood tests have been requested. A variety of devices are available to draw blood into evacuated tubes.

- ProGuard II™ Safety Needle Holder,

  MONOJECT™ ANGEL WING™ Blood Collection Sets with Needle Holder,

  MONOJECT™ ANGEL WING™ Blood Collection/Infusion Sets with Female Luer,

  MONOJECT™ ANGEL WING™ Blood Collection/Infusion Sets with Multi-Sample Luer Adapter,

  ANGEL WING™ Blood Collection Assembly with MONOJECT BLUNTIP™ Safety I.V. Access Cannula,

  ANGEL WING™ Luer Lock Collection Set,

  MONOJECT™ ANGEL WING™ Multi-Sample Collection Sets-Male; Covidien, www.kendallhealthcare.com

  VACUETTE® VISIO PLUS Blood Collection Needle,

  VACUETTE® Safety Tube Holders,

  MiniCollect Capillary Blood Collection System;

  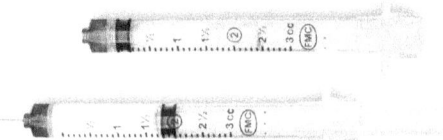

  Greiner Bio One; www.gbo.com/preanalytics

- Vacutainer Eclipse Blood Collection Needle,

  Vacutainer® Push Button Blood Collection Set,

  Vacutainer® Safety-Lok™ Blood Collection Set,

  Eclipse Safety Shielding Blood Collection Needle, One Use Stackable Holder,

  Vacutainer Passive Shielding Blood Collection Needle with Integrated Blood Tube Holder,

  Vacutainer® Eclipse™ Blood Collection Needle,

  Vacutainer® Push Button Collection Set,

  BD Vacutainer Flashback Needle; BD, www.bd.com

- VanishPoint Blood Collection Tube Holder (needle-retracting tube holder with back-end needle protection); Retractable Technologies, www.vanishpoint.com
- One Stick Y extension set with Volumeter, One Stick LLC, www.1stick.com
- Punctur-Guard Blood Collection Needle; Gaven Medical; www.gavenmedical.com

Blood Culture Bottles

A blood culture is a laboratory test in which blood is injected into bottles of culture media to determine whether microorganisms have invaded the patient's bloodstream. These blood cultures are ordered as a set consisting of two bottles, one that is an aerobic bottle and one that is an anaerobic bottle. A blood culture is done when a person has symptoms of a blood infection or bacteremia. Blood is withdrawn from the person and is then tested in a laboratory to find and identify any microorganism present and growing in the blood. This allows the physician to prescribe antibiotics if a microorganism is found. Blood is drawn from a person suspected of blood infection and is put directly into a blood culture bottle containing a nutritional broth. Some culture bottles allow clinicians to use safety needled products in transferring the blood.

- BD BACTEC™/F Blood Culture Procedural Trays; BD, www.bd.com .
- WorkSafe™ Blood Culture Kit; bioMérieux Inc., www.biomerieux-usa.com

Blood Culture Bottle Sample Introduction
These products are used to collect samples into vacuum blood culture bottles for bacterial detection and test tubes for laboratory tests.

- MONOJECT™ ANGEL WING™ BacT/ALERT™* Blood Collection Device-Male,

  MONOJECT™ ANGEL WING™ BacT/ALERT™* Transfer Device-Female Tyco Healthcare/Kendall, www.kendallsharpsafety.com

- ITL Samplok® Sampling Kit, Samplok® Adapter Cap; ITL,www.itlcorporation.com/ssk.php
- Safety Shield For Blood Culture Bottles; Innovative Laboratory Acrylics;www.innovativelabacrylics.com/products/pages/lsshield.html

Blood Donor Needles
Blood donor needles transfers blood from a blood donor into donor bags. Following the blood donation the needle is retracted or shielded to prevent needlestick injuries.

- TERUFLEX® Blood Bags with Blood Sampling Arm® and Donor*Care*® Needle Guard, Terumo, www.terumotransfusion.com/

Blood Filtration Set
Blood filtration set designed for the neonatal infusion of frequently administered small volumes of blood, blood components and other fluids subject to micro filtration. The filtration set replaces a needle filter.

- Hemo-Nate® blood filtration set, Utah Medical Products, Inc;www.utahmed.com/hemonate.htm

Blood Slide Preparation Devices
These products eliminate the need to remove the stopper from the blood tube. The old and potentially dangerous method to prepare differential slides was to take two glass slides, open a blood tube by removing its cap, place a drop of blood onto one of the slides and then place one slide against the other one. New safety products can eliminate the potential of exposure to bloodborne pathogens and without the risk of broken glass or blood splatter.

- Diff-Safe Blood Dispenser; Alpha Scientific Corp., www.alpha-scientific.com
- Haemo-Diff Blood Smear; Sarstedt, www.sarstedt.com
- H-Pette Slide Preparation Device; Helena Laboratories,www.helena.com/miscPlastics.htm

Blood Splash Protection
OSHA has recommended that healthcare workers protect themselves from biohazardous splashes, aerosols, and sprays. One method of doing this is by using transparent shields that can limit bloodborne pathogen exposures.

- Face-it™ Shields; Onyx Medical; www.onyzmedical.com
- LSS Laboratory Safety Shield;; Innovative Laboratory Acrylics;www.innovativelabacrylics.com/products/pages/lsshield.html
- Magni-Guard; Advanced Medical Innovations; www.amiwelisten.com

Blood Transfer Devices
Blood can sometime need to be transferred from a syringe draw to an evacuated tube. Safety products can be used to eliminate sharps and bloodborne pathogen exposure during this process.

- BD Vacutainer® Blood Transfer Device; BD, www.bd.com
- MONOJECT™ ANGEL WING™ Multi-Sample Transfer Sets - Male; Covidien, www.kendallhealthcare.com
- Blood Transfer Device; Greiner Bio-One,www.gbo.com/preanalytics
- BLOOD TUBE HOLDER & SHIELD FOR TRANSFER OF BLOOD FROM SYRINGE TO VACUUM TUBE; Innovative Laboratory Acrylics;www.innovativelabacrylics.com/products/pages/bloodtube.html

Blunt Cannula Needles
Blunt cannula needles can be used in a variety of settings where a cannula is needed but where a sharp one is not required.

- Blunt Cannula Needle, AliMed, www.alimed.com
- Blunt Plastic Cannula, BD Q-Syte Closed Luer Access Septum Port,; BD Twinpak Dual Cannula Device; BDI www.bd.com
- Safeline Split System; B Braun Medical; www.bbraunusa.com/index.html?

Blunt Suture Needles

Blunt needle cannula complies with OSHA Bloodborne Standard for Engineering Controls. Blunt needles can be used to access pre-pierced ports, and single or multi-dose drug vials. Use of these products can increase safety and ease of use by decreasing the number of steps required to draw and deliver intravenous fluids.

- Auto Suture™ENDO STITCH™ 10 mm Suturing Device, PROTECT•POINT™ Blunt Point Needles; U.S. Surgical, www.syneture.com
- Ethiguard Blunt Point; Ethicon, Inc., www.ethicon.com

Bodily Fluid Waste Disposal

In the past, hazardous blood wastes from angiographic catheterizations were "squirted" into an open basin creating a messy, potentially infection problem for clinicians and those required to clean up after the case. Closed waste basins provide a safer alternative and minimize exposure to staff.

- Aspen Basin; Argon Medical Devices, www.argonmedical.com
- BackStop®, BackStop + ®, MiniStop®; Merit Medical, www.merit.com
- SplashStop™ (fluid waste) collection container; Deroyal, www.deroyal.com
- SplashStop™ (fluid waste) collection container; Alimed; www.alimed.com

Bone Marrow Biopsy Needle Kits

Bone marrow biospy needle kits provide all of the components necessary to acquire bone marrow aspirate with safety components included in the kit.

- Kendall® GOLDENBERG SNARECOIL™* Bone Marrow Biopsy and Aspiration Trays with Safety Components,

- MONOJECT™ Bone Marrow Aspiration Trays with Rosenthal Type Needle with Safety Components; Covidien,www.kendallhealthcare.com

Bone Marrow Collection Systems

Closed system that allows for the collection of bone marrow aspirates without healthcare worker exposure.

- Bone Marrow Collection System with Sealed Collection Bag; BioAccess,www.bioaccess.com

Bone Mill, Disposable

Bone mills are used to grind bone to be used for spinal fusion, orthopedic reconstruction, and maxillofacial procedures. These procedures expose health-care workers to sharps injuries. A disposable bone mill can eliminate exposure to sharp injuries for hospital staff, as well as cross-contamination for patients and OR personnel. Since the disposable mill is thrown away after each procedure, there is no risk for blood-borne pathogen exposure.

- Bone Shark Disposable Bone Mill; Medical Innovators, www.medicalinnovators.net

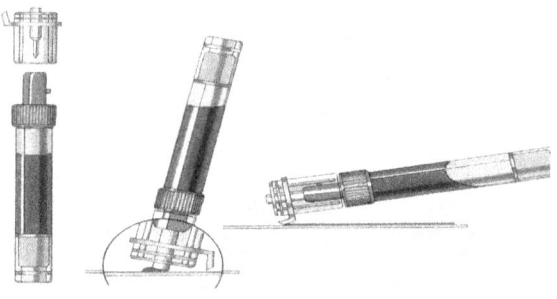

Continue your journey at

www.MedicalSafetyBook.com

Go ahead and order device evaluation samples and literature. Start your device evaluations now.

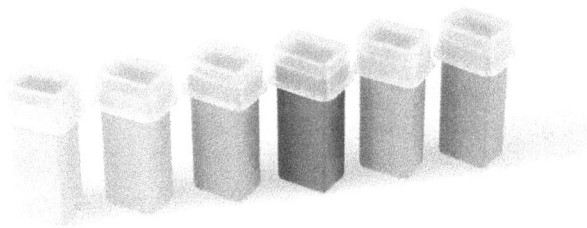

www.ingramcontent.com/pod-product-compliance
Lightning Source LLC
Chambersburg PA
CBHW081449170526
45166CB00008B/2373